Extreme Caregiving

Extreme Caregiving
The Moral Work of Raising Children with Special Needs

LISA FREITAG

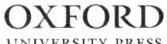

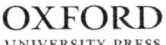

Oxford University Press is a department of the University of Oxford. It furthers
the University's objective of excellence in research, scholarship, and education
by publishing worldwide. Oxford is a registered trade mark of Oxford University
Press in the UK and certain other countries.

Published in the United States of America by Oxford University Press
198 Madison Avenue, New York, NY 10016, United States of America.

© Oxford University Press 2018

All rights reserved. No part of this publication may be reproduced, stored in
a retrieval system, or transmitted, in any form or by any means, without the
prior permission in writing of Oxford University Press, or as expressly permitted
by law, by license, or under terms agreed with the appropriate reproduction
rights organization. Inquiries concerning reproduction outside the scope of the
above should be sent to the Rights Department, Oxford University Press, at the
address above.

You must not circulate this work in any other form
and you must impose this same condition on any acquirer.

Library of Congress Cataloging-in-Publication Data
Names: Freitag, Lisa, author.
Title: Extreme caregiving : the moral work of raising children with special needs /
Lisa Freitag.
Description: New York, NY : Oxford University Press, [2018] |
Includes bibliographical references and index.
Identifiers: LCCN 2017016866 (print) | LCCN 2017018958 (ebook) |
ISBN 9780190491796 (online course) | ISBN 9780190491802 (updf) |
ISBN 9780190491819 (epub) | ISBN 9780190491789 (pbk. : alk. paper)
Subjects: LCSH: Children with disabilities—Care. | Parents of children with disabilities.
Classification: LCC RJ138 (ebook) | LCC RJ138 .F74 2018 (print) |
DDC 362.4083—dc23
LC record available at https://lccn.loc.gov/2017016866

9 8 7 6 5 4 3 2 1
Printed by WebCom, Inc., Canada

*For my mother, Elizabeth Rush Freitag,
pioneer in extreme caregiving*

CONTENTS

Preface ix
Acknowledgments xxi

CHAPTER 1 Introduction   1
CHAPTER 2 Defining Extreme Caregiving   8
CHAPTER 3 Hard Labor   32
CHAPTER 4 Narrative and the Phases of Care   64
CHAPTER 5 Attentiveness and Responsibility: The Invisible Work of Care   94
CHAPTER 6 Competence   124
CHAPTER 7 Responsiveness   157
CHAPTER 8 Holding the Future   192
CHAPTER 9 Conclusion: Caring With   222

References 233
Index 241

PREFACE

Not in Holland

I discovered Emily Perl Kingsley's famous essay, "Welcome to Holland," almost twenty years ago, on the side of the refrigerator at my friend Annette's house. It was printed on a plain white sheet of paper, held in place by four heart-shaped magnets. Someone had decorated the edges with cutesy tulips, wooden shoes, and windmills. The paper was a bit wrinkled and torn, like it had been removed and consulted during many stressful times. Between the windmills were splashes of pink stains the exact color of amoxicillin. It clearly had been there a while.

It is no wonder that I hadn't noticed it before. Annette had a very crowded refrigerator; a collage of the usual photographs of relatives, postcards from friends, and projects painted by Annette's son and youngest daughter, both still in elementary school. But the largest portion of the fridge was taken up by the middle child and oldest daughter, Savannah, who was then about six years old. There were a few photos, of course, but most of the fridge door was filled with notebook paper meticulously printed with schedules, lists, and instructions. One sheet held the name, phone number, and specialty of all of Savannah's doctors, about twelve of them, along with a brief description of the sort of emergency each of them might handle. Another held a chart of all of Savvy's medications—a number that fluctuated between eight and fourteen—complete with dosage in milliliters, a description of its effects, and a spread sheet to be filled in each time the medication was given. In the center was a large calendar filled with dates of doctor and therapy appointments, and a much-crossed-out schedule of available home health care workers.

At the time, the essay had been circulating for about ten years, passed from parent to parent. It has become more popular since then and continues to be a feature on the bulletin boards of pediatric specialty clinics and on innumerable parent support websites. It is even referred to in the title of a 2008 memoir about raising a son with Down syndrome by Jennifer Groneberg, which is called *Road Map to Holland*.

In the essay, Kingsley uses a metaphor of going on a trip to explain the experience of preparing for the birth of a child. Most parents, she says, expect to be going to Italy. They read the guidebooks, learn a couple words of Italian, and prepare as well as they can, all the while anticipating the many wonders of Italy. But when a child is born with a disability, the trip has not gone as expected. Instead of Italy, she says, your plane lands in Holland. You might feel disappointment, or even grief, but Holland is not a bad place. It's just not what you expected. And, after you've been there a while, you realize that Holland has its own delights. You merely must be willing to accept that you will be seeing windmills and tulips instead of the Coliseum, and willing to accept the fact that everyone else who wanted to go to Italy got there as planned.

Though Kingsley's essay is quite short, it took me a while to read it. Annette's house was in its usual state of exhausting, barely controlled chaos. I was doing the dinner dishes, which, since we always used paper plates, mostly involved cleaning the many tubes and syringes by which Savvy received her numerous medications. I read the first part of the essay while rinsing. In the middle of the sixth or seventh line, Savvy climbed onto the couch next to her sister and tangled her fingers in her hair. The resulting screams kept all of us busy for a bit. Nothing ever went uninterrupted for more than thirty seconds at Annette's house.

I had, a few years earlier, been one of the doctors on Annette's list, though the lowliest one. I was only a general pediatrician, charged with giving baby shots and sometimes deciding which of the specialists to call for illnesses. One of Savvy's pediatric cardiologists had referred her to me because, I suspected, I had shown some ability to recognize the difference between congestive heart failure and a cold in an infant, which is not as easy as it ought to be. At that point, she was two-and-one-half months old and was leaving the hospital for the first time. She'd had lots of problems during her months in the neonatal intensive care unit (NICU), involving almost every bodily system, though the syndrome that caused them had not been identified. The worst problem was several unexplained calcifications in her heart muscles, some of which were in a position to interrupt her heartbeat. She had episodes of unstoppable arrhythmia leading to heart failure but was finally stabilized on two new medications, both of which were still experimental in children. The combination was the only thing that had worked. I got the impression from the cardiologist that he did not expect Savvy to survive.

I did not visit Annette during those first months, but I have stood by others during that nightmarish time in the NICU. I've watched as plans for a happy, timely discharge from the hospital turn into bedside vigils that can last for days, then weeks, then months. Life for these parents turns into a series of encounters with previously unsuspected and unknown details, with hope or despair hanging day-to-day on miniscule changes in ventilator settings or potassium levels or blood gas measurements. Meanwhile, that anticipated homecoming, surrounded by balloons and flowers and smiles, recedes into a distant, unattainable dream.

In the essay, the trip to Holland is easy: a sudden and unexpected arrival in a different country. Certainly, Annette had set off for Italy yet had not reached there. But on the way, she'd spent months in the limbo of Savannah's bedside in the NICU. She would have recognized that the expected trip to parenthood was not going as planned. Kingsley's metaphorical trip to Italy had been, at best, seriously delayed. Perhaps the plane was stuck at the airport, maybe still sitting on the runway. Those months in the hospital were ever so much more uncomfortable than an airport, and on every trip to and from the NICU, there was the possibility of passing the joyous train of someone else, some other family, who was about to successfully disembark in Italy.

Parents who come to the place Kingsley calls Holland do not arrive all at once, but in long, anxious stages. Many parents live suspended, as Annette did, between one medical crisis and the next, hoping only that their child will live to arrive anywhere. Most of them don't realize how different that place will be until they finally arrive at that long-awaited day when their child is discharged. The hospital staff sends them off with smiles and waves, along with all the baby supplies brought in to make the NICU seem more livable. In those months, both flowers and balloons have wilted, but you can gather an awful lot of plushie toys. Annette also took with her an apnea monitor, an oxygen tank, prescriptions for fourteen medications, and the equipment needed to give continuous G-tube feedings, as well as to perform emergency CPR. Finally home with Savannah and her roomful of medical equipment, she found that her house now had all the comforts of a hospital, but considerably less staff.

I'm sure that Annette received the necessary training in the use of home medical equipment, but I, at least, had not thought about what her home might look like with all that stuff. I saw Savannah's bedroom several months after she'd arrived home, at a combination house call and birthday party. There had been an attempt, at one point, to create a Disney-themed baby girl's room. The walls were painted yellow to match a poster of Minnie Mouse. A Little Mermaid mobile had been taken down, likely because it was in the way, and was collapsed on top of a pile of medical tubing, rubber gloves, and protective pads. The matching lamp was partly hidden by the apnea monitor and the emergency bag and mask, ready for use in case Savvy actually stopped breathing. The oxygen tank was on the floor, dwarfed by the IV stand, which held a translucent bag of formula and the pump that regulated its flow down the tube leading to Savvy's stomach. The obligatory comfy rocking chair, which suburban mothers at that time considered a necessary adjunct to breastfeeding, was occupied by a young woman, a nursing student at the local community college. She was one of many women Annette hired and paid to watch Savannah overnight, in the hopes of getting some sleep herself. Savannah, sleeping in the crib, was very hard to see.

Over the next few years, I saw Savvy every few months, whenever a general pediatric visit was necessary on Annette's complicated schedule. I ordered Savvy's baby shots and sent her back to the children's hospital ICU when the usual childhood illnesses caused her to go into heart failure. She spent nearly one-third of her first year in the hospital. I prescribed many of the medications listed on the refrigerator door and provided refills of others. I both looked forward to and dreaded visits, because I enjoyed seeing Savannah and Annette, but their visits never failed to set my schedule behind by at least an hour. There was never enough time to do everything that Annette clearly needed from me. I thought I was working hard but rarely thought about how hard Annette must work to carry out my orders.

When Savvy was six, I moved to another clinic where I could practice part time, and where the administrators told me that a child as complex as Savannah could not be seen. Happily, that left me free to accept Annette's invitation of play dates with my son and her other two children, only a few years apart in age. My son quickly became friends with both Annette's son and youngest daughter, and our visits became frequent.

Savannah never played with the others. By then, she could walk, and get into things, but showed no interest in the games and books and videos the others shared. She had finally gotten rid of the oxygen tank and most of the heart medicines, but the touch of food near her mouth made her cry and gag, so she still needed tube feedings. Dinners were a complicated affair, beginning with an attempt to overcome Savvy's oral aversion by touching her mouth with tiny amounts of baby food. After any vomiting had been dealt with, Savvy got a twenty-minute feeding of formula mixed with vitamins, straight into her stomach via her G-tube. Not wanting to restrain her during this time, Annette would follow her around the house, holding the end of the tube high and pouring little bits at a time into the giant syringe at the top. When they wandered back through the kitchen, Annette would get a bite or two of her own meal.

Savvy couldn't talk either. She communicated by a limited number of signs, and by crying or laughing. She loved the sound of car horns, and if, at the beginning and end of a car ride, you forgot to honk the horn, she would moan in protest, then laugh and clap enthusiastically when you remembered. She never tired of this game. When she was not in the car, the game of keeping her occupied was harder. Even when she was not being fed, Annette still followed Savvy around the house, putting away the things she scattered, talking to her, and giving her a different toy every time she cried. It was impossible to tell what Savvy wanted, only that she wanted something, and Annette never gave up the attempt to find just the right combination. If she guessed wrong, Savvy would shift from whining to screaming. If she guessed right, Savvy would reward her with laughter and, maybe, a few minutes of peace.

By the time I found the essay on her refrigerator door, Annette would have known that she wasn't in Italy and wasn't ever going to get there. Kingsley's essay, lovingly posted on the refrigerator door and showing signs of much use, must have provided enormous reassurance and validation. Annette hadn't gotten to Italy with Savvy, but the place that she had arrived in was, according to Kingsley, "just a different place . . . slower paced [and] less flashy than Italy." More importantly, that place had its own different rewards—windmills, tulips, and Rembrandts—which were available once she was able to move past the disappointment.

Annette had lived for some time with the grief that comes with a loss of something expected but not attained—that normal dream child, Italy. According to Kingsley, the pain of losing Italy will "never, ever, ever, go away." That loss seemed often to be there in the background. We had many hours of conversations, multiply interrupted, of course, in which Annette told me, and herself, that everything was going to be fine. She hung her hopes for a more normal life on overcoming the current medical crisis, or on anticipated medication changes, or on new school programs or therapies. Yet, according to the essay, she was supposed to be able to just get over any difficulties, simply by recognizing that where she'd ended up was merely a different place, happily called Holland.

I've been to Holland, and it is a wonderful place. There are, indeed, windmills and tulips and Rembrandts. Holland also has clearly marked intersections and virtually no language barrier. It has plenty of sleep, few interruptions, and no need to hire a guide, let alone your own home health care team. Many people, including me, actually prefer Holland over Italy and travel there intentionally. But very few people go to Kingsley's metaphorical Holland on purpose; they land there by accident. As I finished washing the endless pile of plastic tubes and syringes, I thought, I don't know where we are, but it isn't Holland.

Annette's place was nothing like Holland. This new place held a confusing array of diagnoses, medications, and procedures, each of which had its own description in the unfamiliar language of medicine. The only guidance through this was provided by an equally confusing array of professionals. The stakes for failure were exorbitantly high—the life of a child, no less—and following the directions required so much work. The very idea that someone could attempt to reassure Annette by comparing this experience to nothing more than a detour to Holland seemed appallingly naive, almost insulting.

I have also been a visitor to the place that Kinglsey calls Holland. I had grown up there, more or less. My arrival began in 1960 when my brother Paul was born, the second of twins, at 32 weeks. He spent his first month in the 1960 equivalent of a NICU, where not much was available in the way of treatment. Then he was sent home, limp, unmoving, and unable to suck from a bottle. My mother never found out how they fed him in the hospital. She fed him with an eye dropper, every two hours, for over a year.

Throughout his first year, doctors told my mother that there was absolutely nothing wrong with him, but at fourteen months it could no longer be denied. Paul was still not holding his head up, and he was just beginning to be able to down a four-ounce bottle in less than an hour. In a reversal of their previous assessment, the doctors decided that, in fact, something was terribly wrong, and, as a result, he would never be able to walk or talk. My parents were then advised to place him in an institution. This they refused to do, though they said later they had no idea why they did not follow the recommendation. It was years before the horrific conditions at Pennhurst, our local institution, were revealed, and a decade before the experiments at Willowbrook were publicized. I was five, way too young to know what a momentous decision they had made for all of us.

I was also too young to recognize that my mother had spent every other hour, round the clock, during that first year just feeding Paul, one drop at a time. These days, a baby like Paul would be given a feeding tube just like

Savannah's, a procedure that my mother finds both horrifying and indicative of laziness on the part of mothers of my generation. She is incorrect about that. I am not convinced that a G-tube would have reduced her caregiving time. It certainly was not much of a time-saver for Annette. But, unlike Paul, without the tube Savannah could not have been fed at all.

Over the years, even as Paul's development improved, our family life revolved increasingly around Paul's care. My mother protected us from most of the feeding and diapering and bathing, but we were encouraged to take part in what passed for education and physical therapy for him. We celebrated every miniscule step in his slow developmental gains, though I admit that my own pride in his accomplishments was tinged with cynicism. We have home movies of me, my sister, and Paul's twin brother Walter pretending to have fun in the living room with a set of parallel bars, constructed by my father to teach Paul to walk. My techie father spliced onto this later footage of us helping Paul to grab the bars, and then, incredibly, pull himself along them, walking. He was seven.

I did not go to medical school thinking, or even hoping, I would be able to cure my brother. I did not go into pediatrics because I thought I would be able to learn what had happened to cause his problems. Nor did I expect to be able to keep it from happening to other kids. Eventually though I did form an idea of what had happened. His disability is consistent with what is now called hypoxic-ischemic encephalopathy, lack of oxygen at the time of delivery causing damage to the brain. It is not uncommon in prematurity or in difficult deliveries, both of which occurred with my brother. It is possible that, if my mother had had a Caesarian, Paul would have had a very different life. So would have we all.

According to Kingsley, that life would have merely been different, not necessarily better or worse. Perhaps she is right. We can't know that any of us, including Paul, would have been more or less happy, accomplished more or less, or been better or worse people. Maybe I wouldn't have gone to medical school. Maybe medical school wasn't the best thing for me. The only thing I'm sure of is that life with Paul provided a visible and constant reminder that life does not always go as expected. My cynicism in the face of Kingsley's essay may stem from learning at a very early age that Italy is not guaranteed for anyone.

In medical school, I learned the language that is spoken in this country that is neither Italy nor Holland. I became fluent in the multisyllabic words that are flung about in the describing and diagnosing of diseases. It is likely easier to learn them when they are abstract words applied to other people, and when their specific and often dire meanings are not being used to identify the things that your child might die of. And I became part of the team that keeps kids from dying of those things, and sends them home to their grateful but unsuspecting families.

Despite having grown up there and being versed in the language, I did not know much about the country to which Savannah's birth had exiled Annette. As her pediatrician, I blithely ordered yet another medication, never counting how many there were or thinking about how long it might take to measure and administer them all. I ordered more tests and recommended more visits to specialists, never adding up just how long these meant in hours spent for Annette. I did know that she'd had to abandon completing her PhD in social work in order to take care of Savannah. My mother had given up a career as well, though in the sixties no one ever really expected her to have one. But it wasn't until I started spending time at Annette's house that I realized just how far away the country in which they both lived was.

If it wasn't Holland, then where was it? Growing up, I would have guessed that it was somewhere bleak and horrible; where everyone works dawn to dusk with no sleep doing something incredibly boring and pointless. But, of course, that is unfair. Kingsley says, "The important thing is that they haven't taken you to a horrible, disgusting, filthy place, full of pestilence, famine and disease. It's just a different place." Annette's place was chaotic and exhausting, but the work was neither dangerous nor disgusting. There were times when the work was tedious, but it was never pointless. The center of that work, grounded in her steadfast love and care for Savannah, was one of the joys to be discovered there. Kingsley is correct that the place she calls Holland is not without rewards.

Though my family did many things right, we did indeed miss this important aspect. Or at least I did. For me, Paul's disability was totally about loss. I always thought of Paul in terms of who he could have been, not who he was. My celebration of his accomplishments, coming slowly but regularly, was always clouded by a touch of grief or anger for the things he would never do: read a book, make proper change at the grocery store, live independently.

Kingsley would say that we were wasting time mourning Italy and thus unable to recognize the good things we had where we were. And she would be at least partly right. We did recognize Paul as an important member of our family, and we celebrated the gains he made to the best of our ability. But we were unable to ignore the difficulties. We were comparing Paul to a person that we thought he could have been, if only the brain injury at birth had not taken him away. There was no way to properly mourn this loss, no social means to express it, and no shared ceremony to encompass it. Though it was not quantifiable, our loss was nonetheless real and not so easily dismissed.

Recognizing the tension between loss and gain is one of the difficulties in living in that place that isn't Holland. Linda is the mother of Samuel, who was diagnosed with Cornelia DeLang syndrome (CDLS), a cluster of problems that, according to my medical school textbooks from the 1980s, are usually fatal by age five or so. A prenatal ultrasound at eight months showed that parts of his brain were missing and that he had a heart defect that would require multiple open-heart surgeries, beginning right after birth. The physician thought that he was unlikely to survive the surgeries and advised Linda to forgo treatment and let him die, but she decided instead to give him whatever life he could have. Samuel was born with CDLS, with its many associated disabilities, but his heart defects were not as bad as they looked. He had a single successful operation when he was one week old, which corrected the problem, though he may need some follow-up procedures as he grows.

At eight years, Samuel was functioning at the level of a two-year-old. Like Annette, Linda had to quit her job and work long hours to take care of him. Samuel was learning to talk, a fascinating process which stretched out stages of development that usually last a few weeks, at most, over several years. It took him two years to go from incoherent single syllables to two-word phrases that were understandable only if you knew his language. And every step of the way—each ASL sign, each properly pronounced sound, each word found and used—did indeed hold its own joy. It was a struggle for me, and sometimes for Linda, to avoid comparing him to where he ought to be, and grieve. But when you visited Samuel's house, and he greeted you with an imperious "Coa Oo! Sue Oo!" that meant "Coat, Off! Shoes, Off!," which clearly meant "I am totally thrilled you are here, and I want you to stay," it was equally hard not to smile.

Everything that Samuel felt, learned, and did was an addition to his life, not a subtraction from what he might have been. Perhaps this is because Linda had a chance to choose otherwise for him, and thus fully accepted his disability well before birth, but I don't think that is the entire reason. My mother also had a choice; she could have placed Paul in an institution and tried to forget about him as soon as his diagnosis was evident. But she also chose to give him what life she could. Despite the differences in their knowledge when they made the choice, neither was fully prepared for the consequences. Linda was simply a different person, and she was much better than most of my family at recognizing and celebrating the gains.

Though Linda lived by the sentiments of "Welcome to Holland" far better than my family ever managed, she was not entirely comfortable with the essay. She had heard of it, of course—all parents of children with special needs encounter it eventually—but she did not find much comfort in it. Linda's motto, "It is what it is," was posted in a small framed picture at the top of the stairs, and she lived by it in both triumph and tragedy.

Bringing Samuel home from the hospital was, for Linda, like being lost in an alien city, maybe somewhere on an alien planet. (She is not alone in this analogy. Another parent, the father of a girl with severe autism, called the exhausting and chaotic place where he lives "Planet Autism" [Sea, 2003], but autism is far from the only diagnosis in this other world.) It felt like she had been dropped in darkness into an unknown place with no idea how she got there, or where she needed to go, or even if there was somewhere safe to aim for. I can imagine them there, Linda and other parents like her, surrounded by unknown shadowy forms and holding desperately onto their child who has suddenly but not unexpectedly become the most precious person in the world. All they can do at first is stand there, in the middle of a busy intersection, hoping for direction. Those first steps are often dictated by medical attention the child urgently needs. The people around them, mostly medical professionals, are trying to help but speak another language, so it's hard to be sure. But eventually tiny lights come on. Words begin to make sense. Parents begin to make forays into this new, frightening country, one step at a time. Eventually they learn the way from one location to another and gradually piece together a map from the places they find.

Kingsley is correct in her assessment that this new world is not an unlivable place—not a war zone or a post-apocalyptic nightmare. She is correct to point out that there are joys and triumphs. It is a different place, not better or worse than what was expected, as the child is no more or less valued because of their disability. But I think it is much harder to live in that place than in Italy, and the essay trivializes the challenges of living there.

The essay acknowledges that the pain of losing Italy never goes away, but then states that loss must be put aside in order to see the special things available in Holland. "But if you spend your life mourning the fact that you didn't get to Italy, you may never be free to enjoy the very special, the very lovely things about Holland." This underplays the difficulty of maintaining an attitude of positivity and effectively assigns blame to parents who fail to properly recognize and celebrate the joys of Holland. When, in the middle of a sleepless night, or after a behavior setback, or during a medical crisis, parents find themselves longing for Italy, they are supposed to make a better effort to be happy, to insist that they live in a great place called Holland. This is not always possible and may be too much to ask.

Unlike Holland, there is no map of this place. The place itself is unacknowledged, as though it were an alien city. Sane people are unaware of its existence, and the reliability of those who are witnesses to it is questioned. Every parent who is randomly selected to land in this unexplored country seems to discover a slightly different place. In order to describe it, we must acknowledge the frustrations and disappointments and sorrows, as well as the benefits. Any good map must include all of it.

Holland fails for me because it brushes aside many significant difficulties, perhaps making it easier for us to ignore hardships the parents might endure. The place that is not Holland is neither composed of unmitigated loss and hardship nor entirely full of windmills and tulips. It is neither completely dire nor completely wonderful. The gifts that exist in this place are often hard to recognize and sometimes come at great cost. This is a world, as we will come to see, wherein unbearable sorrow and heady joy exist side by side, embodied in the same child.

ACKNOWLEDGMENTS

This book would not exist without Joan Liaschenko, who provided assistance and much-needed support in every phase. She read the manuscript in all its iterations, beginning with rough drafts of a very vague student project. Her door was always open for friendly advice, discussion, encouragement, and, sometimes, tea and cookies. I owe her thanks for everything from suggesting better word choices to gently correcting misunderstandings of feminist ethics. It is a much better book because of her caring. Any remaining mistakes are entirely my own.

I owe many thanks to the caregivers: Sandy, Annette, and Linda, who invited me into their homes and from there into their hearts. Sandy was the first to show me that despite tragedy, life goes on in joy. Annette's forbearance and never-ending hopefulness in the face of hardship helped me recognize the ambiguity inherent in extreme caregiving. Linda taught me patience and acceptance, and the excitement that comes from watching a child make slow progress through developmental phases and sharing the pride of accomplishment at every incremental step.

I suspect they all still have lessons for me. Their kindness throughout the process of writing this book is deeply appreciated. I hope I did not try their patience too much.

Thanks also are due to the faculty and staff at the University of Minnesota Center for Bioethics. They welcomed me as a very nontraditional graduate student and continued to provide assistance even after I had graduated. Special thanks to Mary Faith Marshall who began this project with me, Joan Tronto who helped me dissect her theories, and John Song who was there at the end.

I could not have written this without the assistance of the Brothers of Charity, who have, for the last twenty-five years, taken care of my brother Paul for me. Special thanks go to Brother Mike and to Brother John, who have devoted much of their lives to my brother and who showed me the difference between providing a service and providing care. Thanks also go to my other brother, Walter, who not only is Paul's official guardian but who also as a writer provided much needed editing and advice.

And, of course, thanks and love to my husband Greg, who has stood by me all these years and never complained about my many time-consuming projects.

CHAPTER 1 | Introduction

PARENTS WHO HAVE a child with disabilities find themselves in a different world, which is often foreign to their expectations about raising a child. The exact nature, and possibly the actual existence, of this new country, is contested. Emily Perl Kingsley, in her famous essay "Welcome to Holland" describes it as arriving in Holland rather than Italy, but many see this as an oversimplification of a complicated process. There is no doubt, however, that the arrival of a child with special needs irrevocably alters the lives of the parents. Their life journey has taken a new trajectory into unknown territory. And whether they arrive unexpectedly or intentionally, due to a random accident or planned birth, most of them must construct for themselves a new map of the place where they now live.

To highlight the extraordinary nature of the journey taken by parents of children with special needs, particularly those who are intellectually disabled or require complex medical care in the home, I call the task that they have been given "extreme caregiving." We shall see that, like an extreme sport, extreme caregiving provides both amazing highs and dangerous lows. There are no established rules for this new way of parenting, and often the players have to figure out their own way of doing things. There are also no accepted measurements for either success or failure. And, like an extreme sport, extreme caregiving can be arduous and lonely and is often misunderstood.

Though each family's journey through this place that is neither Italy nor Holland is different, there are similarities in their experiences, creating areas that by necessity appear on many families' maps. It is perhaps not surprising that interactions with the medical system provide many of the most common places visited on the journey taken by extreme caregivers. Almost everyone requires the help of medical providers; an army of doctors, nurses, therapists, teachers, and care workers, all specializing in some aspect of the child. Health care professionals are both the ensurers of the child's survival and the most knowledgeable collaborators in their care.

We will not find much evidence for or documentation of the existence of extreme caregiving in the medical records however. Though the medical chart holds a summary of the child's needs, it provides a very limited picture. It is a story told in test results, lists of diagnoses and medications, consultations from pediatric subspecialists, and hospital discharge summaries. In the days before electronic records, those charts outgrew their manila folders at an alarming rate, and it was not unusual to have a stack of medical records that weighed more than the child. Yet the total amount of care work required is consistently missing from that story, making it difficult to determine the extent of the care tasks that the parents have been assigned. Hints can be found, in transfers to units that offer more intensive care or in statements that the child requires one-to-one nursing, but these are deeply buried in the masses of more important data.

The effect on the parents' lives is likewise missing from this record. There might be an occasional "Social History" note about parental coping abilities or a brief nursing note about parental presence or absence during a shift. The dedication of the parent to the child and the child's health is usually clear, but the actions necessary to carry out that dedication in the home are not. Parents are often handed copies of instructions after doctor visits or hospital stays, but no one notices if these run to dozens of pages that, quite possibly, require around-the-clock actions. When these children's numerous, often complex, medical regimens are administered at home, their care is effectively out of sight, and it is easy for medical providers to overlook the parents who are providing the care they prescribe.

There is evidence to be found, however, in pediatric medicine, ethics, and disability studies literature, all of which have been nibbling around slightly different edges of the territory. Children whose care can be predicted to be complex and time-consuming can be found at the most severe end of a multitude of pediatric conditions. This includes children whose medical problem lists contain numerous items (ten to twenty is not unusual) and children with a single diagnosis that encompasses multiple disabilities. Other children require care work based on the severity of a single problem. Children with severe intellectual disabilities or at the most compromised end of the autism spectrum, for example, can also be predicted to require an enormous amount of care.

Because these children fall across a large number of chronic diseases, syndromes, and diagnoses, and because their medical needs and types of disability vary so widely, those who do require high levels of care have not yet been identified as a distinct group. They are often referred to as "children with special needs," a term I will continue to use for convenience, though it is neither precise nor universally accepted. In fact, they are not all even technically children, as many have grown to adulthood but still require a level of care usually encountered only in infants or small children. Despite these differences in age, diagnosis, and disability, they all have in common an ongoing need for care that is intense, exhausting, and prolonged. Their parents must provide special care, combined with the usual duties of parenting, which are often extended by the child's problems.

And so the first task of this book is to find proof that parents of children with a multitude of different needs are indeed on a similar journey and that there are enough people living in the country they discover that a map can be constructed. I begin in Chapter 2 with a more extensive definition of extreme caregiving. I also review the available academic information on families providing complex home care for their children, and hazard an estimation of both their current numbers and speculate on the way those numbers might change over time.

The next goal is to provide a fuller description of the lives of extreme caregivers. In Chapter 3, I begin to correlate information about extreme caregiving extrapolated from academic studies, with information provided in stories told and written by the parents who live there. I will draw from the stories of the caregivers I introduced in the Preface; from Linda's story, and Annette's, and my mother's. I will retell a few stories that I heard or observed in my pediatric practice. My largest source of information about extreme caregiving is not personal, however. It is from longer narratives: autobiographies and essays written by parents who have dared to expose their feelings—both positive and negative—in books published over the last several decades.

Correlating this information is made more difficult by the changing nature of the work over time. When my brother was born, in 1960, doctors at that time had nothing much to offer him—no feeding therapy, no early child development programs, no genetic testing, and certainly no cure. With the work of caring for him, my parents took on the fight to find or create the things he needed to develop and thrive. It was not an easy task.

Parents today whose children have impairments similar to my brother's are offered a variety of supports that were not available to my parents. They do not have to invent their own physical therapy programs and advocate for the basic right to education, as my parents did. Their children have access to an interwoven system of medical, behavioral, and educational programs. They are supported by an extensive (and expensive) network, which from the outside looks more than sufficient. Yet their work is not any easier. They must keep track of multiple appointments, perform the many recommended home exercises, and ensure that the classroom is meeting their child's unique needs. None of these necessary things are likely to simplify the lives of the parents.

In addition, many parents also have to deal with complex medical problems that were not a problem in the 1960s, simply because children that sick did not survive. Those who did survive, if they required any medical technology, had to remain in professional care facilities. Savannah, whose cardiac arrhythmias responded only to newly developed, experimental medications, likely would not have survived infancy even ten years earlier. She certainly would not have been able to live at home. And Samuel, who has Cornelia DeLange syndrome, survives because of advances in several pediatric subspecialties, which allow his multiple and unique medical problems to be kept at bay. As I write this, Savannah is twenty-three years old and still needs a pediatric cardiologist, endocrinologist, orthopedist, and neurologist, along with a gastroenterologist to monitor her tube feedings. Samuel just passed his eleventh birthday with no sign of slowing down, despite ongoing problems with delayed development, kidney disease, seizures, short stature, and impaired vision. Like numerous kids with special needs, Savannah and Samuel owe their survival to advances in medicine but are sustained day-to-day by their parents' hard work.

When we talk about the ethics of modern medicine, we acknowledge some of the consequences of scientific advances, but we rarely recognize the resulting increased need for care. Likewise, standard discussions of pediatric ethics often overlook the care provided by parents. In Chapter 4, I outline, using a parent narrative, some different ways in which ethical discussions regarding children with special needs have been approached and suggest ways to add consideration of problems that might arise from the need for extreme caregiving. I hope to provide a new framework for analysis of caregiver narratives based on theories advanced by political scientist and care ethicist Joan Tronto.

Advances in medical science have made it possible to present parents with sometimes difficult and terrible decisions. In the literature on pediatric ethics, parents are usually entrusted with the power to make all medical decisions for their dependent child. The common position among pediatricians and ethicists is that parents have a duty to make those decisions entirely in the best interests of the child (Lantos & Kohrman, 1992). There are agreed-upon standards for the things owed to children, and reasonable lists of the things that constitute their best interests (Malek, 2009). The needs of the vulnerable child often are thought to outweigh any preferences the parents might have. Thus, we ask parents to make sometimes difficult medical decisions for their children entirely without regard to the way in which the decision might impact their own lives.

Not all ethicists agree that the family's interests must always be set aside in favor of the patient, however. John Hardwig (1997) makes a case for the importance of paying attention to other voices surrounding the patient. He calls the current form of patient-centered ethics, which requires that we consider only the patient's interests, a form of oppression that effectively silences all other members of the family. He states, "Decisions are made every day that promote the patient's interests at truly staggering costs to the lives of other members of the patient's family. These decisions are routinely made as if families were no more than patient support systems or as if the interests of other members of the family were somehow morally irrelevant" (p. 59). Hardwig is speaking here about caregiving for adult family members. However, many medical decisions in pediatrics likewise impact the lives of both the child with special needs and the parent who is providing for these needs.

I am not suggesting that parents should begin making decisions for their children based on their own needs. However I do wish to point out that in thinking only about the child's interests, we ignore an essential part of the equation. We assign the provision of care for a child with medical and developmental needs, no matter how complex, to the parents, seemingly as a consequence of their parenthood. Our lengthy discussions of the principles behind parental decisions, conducted with very little understanding of the effect those decisions might have on the parents' lives, are not complete.

More importantly, those who ask parents to make difficult decisions do not have an accurate account of the effect home caregiving might have on the parents. Even if we did wish to add concerns about the effect of caregiving for children with special needs on the parents' lives to our ethical equations, accurate information on that effect is very hard to find. I have said there is very little information on the lives of parents caring for children with special needs to be found in the medical records, in pediatric medical research, or even in ethical discussions. Yet, if we wish parents to make informed medical decisions, based in a real understanding of what they are being asked to choose, we must be aware of all the consequences of such decisions. Perhaps we will not find better, more definitive answers, but I do expect to uncover different questions.

The final goal of this book is to examine some of the problem spots on the map, the places where most, or all, extreme caregivers encounter difficulties. These are the places where a moral compass might need to focus its attention. In the final chapters, we will review some of the aspects of extreme caregiving that are revealed by analyzing parent narratives through the lens of Tronto's phases of care. In each phase, parents encounter a different set of moral challenges. Chapter 5 deals with the consequences of the heightened levels of attentiveness and responsibility that extreme caregiving places on parents. Chapter 6 begins to explore our expectations for parental competence in medical caregiving at home and our current all-or-none methods of responding to the parent who cannot provide adequate care. Chapter 7 is based on the responsiveness inherent in good caregiving. We will analyze the intense relationship that develops between the extreme caregiving parent and the dependent child, concentrating on the enormous ethical responsibility inherent in upholding a unique identity for a child with developmental delays.

In Chapter 8, I return to my parents' stories, telling the last parts of their caregiving journey. Worry about the future is a constant thread through narratives by extreme caregivers. The few narratives available that mention older people with more severe intellectual disabilities or autism are, for the most part, negative. Yet my parents created for my brother a valued life full of happiness and purpose. We will begin to assemble an idea of the things that are necessary to create this future, in hope of extending it to the children growing up today. I believe their parents need to know it is possible.

We will, at the very least, come to recognize the extent of our ignorance about special needs parenting. We do not know if raising children with special needs poses an additional burden, either physical or emotional, on the parent. We do not question the assumption that the provision of extreme care should as a matter of course fall on any parents who happen to have a child with multiple disabilities. We do not know if the tasks involved are too complex or too demanding for a single set of parents to carry out. No one is even trying to measure the amount of work being done, and extreme caregiving remains essentially invisible to our medical system and in our society.

My intent is to align the understanding of health care professionals with the reality of these parents' lives, so that everyone can begin to recognize where they have arrived. Stories of frustration, confusion, and even betrayal by the medical system are common features on the map of this new place. Of course, most health care professionals are trying their best to be helpful but, like me seeing Savannah in my pediatric clinic, they see only a very small part of the situation. Medicine defines the territory of this alien world, and if we wish to be adequate guides for parents, we must understand what it is like to live there. Comforting images of Holland may make everyone feel better, but feeling better is not always what is needed.

This book is not meant to provide a thorough guidebook for parents, though it may do that to some extent, but to provide an understanding for everyone who works with these families. For our care to truly be effective, we must have a fuller understanding of the journey on which these parents have unexpectedly embarked. We must acknowledge the full extent of the mapless territory, which is neither Italy nor Holland, that they now must explore. This book is for those of us—from friends and family, to the village of involved health care professionals and nonprofessionals—who wish to be a help rather than another frustrating detour in their journey.

I summarize what is known, or can be guessed, about the unique challenges in raising children with special needs from a variety of medical sources, add to that knowledge by listening to the words of parent caregivers, and then speculate on what this task might mean for the parent caregiver and, ultimately, the child. I believe that a good, hard look at the lives of the parents of children with special needs—including the trials as well as the triumphs—will uncover a need to question many of our current assumptions and attitudes.

I suspect that parents taking care of children with special needs at home have been asked to sacrifice much to the best interests of their child. That they seemingly do so willingly, and even find joy in it, does not make their sacrifice any less imposing.

CHAPTER 2 | Defining Extreme Caregiving

IN HIS MEMOIR *The Boy in the Moon: A Father's Journey to Understand His Extraordinary Son*, Ian Brown, writes:

> Until recently, no one . . . was willing to admit that a child could be loved and still be too difficult to be cared for by his or her parents. Because until twenty years ago, children this medically complex didn't exist. They didn't survive. High-tech medicine has created a new strain of human beings who require superhuman care. Society has yet to acknowledge this reality, especially at a practical level. (2011, pp. 95–96)

Brown is the father of one of those medically complex children whose survival is made possible by recent advances in medicine. As medical providers, or even as consumers of the benefits of modern medicine, it is easy to congratulate ourselves on the collective scientific prowess that enabled this extraordinary survival, and let the story end there. We usually fail to acknowledge that for many of these children survival does not guarantee typical health and development. They often have multisystemic, evolving medical problems that continue to affect their health or even threaten their lives. They also are frequently left with multiple disabilities, causing significant delays in growth and development.

We forget that, sometimes, these children's lives are maintained, not only through specialized medical care, but also by constant vigilance and elaborate home care. The families of the children who represent that "new strain of human beings," benefit enormously from that survival but often also pay a high price for it. Brown is all too aware of the amount of care that can be required, having provided it for his son for thirteen years of physically intense days and sleepless nights. Brown's care for his son was indeed a superhuman undertaking.

We will return later to Ian Brown and what we can learn from his writing about his relationship to his son. For now, the important thing is his assertion that we as a society, both within the medical system and in general, have failed to recognize the reality of providing care for children with special needs. High-tech medicine, by enabling the survival of medically complex children, has implicitly assumed some responsibility for their lives. But many clinicians, while providing excellent medical care, lack an understanding of the work of caregiving, and therefore cannot fully support the endeavor of raising them as loved human beings.

Like other care work, the caregiving that the parents and families of these children provide is largely unrecognized. Their children are visible in schools and communities, but the work done at home is not always apparent. Even the physicians and hospitals who provide medical care often do not realize the extent or the practical consequences of the care they prescribe. This is a problem that can be expected to worsen as medical care becomes more constrained by time and more fragmented by specialty.

We have also seen that there are competing narratives about the responsibilities of the parent toward the multiply disabled child. We saw the most basic extremes of those stories in the Preface. On one hand, there is the narrative of living in Holland, where having a child with disabilities is likened to an unexpected detour that, once accepted, becomes wonderful. The opposite is the story my parents were told when they were advised to institutionalize my brother. That story says that raising a child with special needs is dire—an endless round of work with very little gain. We return to these narratives later, as their implications about the value of the child with disabilities and the additional burdens they place on the parents are significant.

I have said that, for pediatric medicine, understanding the journey these parents make is essential. This is, in part, because the parents become the voice of the child and as such become the acknowledged custodians of the child's best interests. More importantly, they are the people who are most significant in the child's life, who must receive the medical care plan and turn it into action, and who must live intimately with the consequences of any decisions. The parents' story is so entwined with the child's that any medical decision made must take the parents' experience of the child's illness into account.

The parents of children with complex medical needs or intellectual disabilities, like my parents, often become vocal advocates for their children. But they rarely stop to pay attention to their own needs. Their own lives are often put aside by the urgent necessity of meeting their child's needs.

Perhaps they are too busy with the endless round of caregiving to think about the superhuman work they are doing. They rarely have time to think about, let alone tell, their own stories. Yet their stories need to be told.

The parents who are willing to tell this story are writing from a relatively unexplored land, where they have been assigned a new and difficult role, that of extreme caregiver. They may indeed report interesting and even wonderful things about living there. But to ignore these parents when they relate stories of hardship essentially silences their voices. Their narratives, I believe, hold an important description of the hidden ethical and emotional consequences of the extreme caregiving relationship. We must stand back and listen to their report from the place that is not Holland.

In this chapter, we will begin with a definition of extreme caregiving, and how the concept arose from early care ethics theories, particularly Eva Feder Kittay's examination of extreme dependency. It is necessary to examine the ways in which extreme caregiving might differ from both typical parenting and from professional caregiving. Since extreme caregiving is often needed in situations ranging from total dependency to multiple additional care needs, we must discuss its most important aspects; the complexity, prolonged duration, relentlessness, and intimacy of the care that must be provided.

Next is a brief foray into medical literature to establish working definitions from the medical language of disability. Any discourse about children with disabilities is hampered by the absence, in the medical literature and elsewhere, of an accurate assessment of level of disability. Indeed, it is likely not possible to arrive at a single scale of "disability," since the range of potential diagnoses and their resulting impairments is enormous. Yet we must realize that the term "special needs" encompasses a broad range of abilities and is not backed by any sort of measurement of need for caregiving. I attempt to briefly summarize the way in which disability is measured in pediatrics and provide my own evaluation of the sorts of caregiving needs that might add up to extreme "special needs."

The chapter ends with an estimation of the numbers of children requiring extreme caregiving, and the effect that pushing the boundaries of medicine might have in the future. The need for extreme caregiving is not a rare or unusual circumstance. But, since the children who require extreme caregiving cross so many boundaries of diagnosis and types of medical need, it is difficult to determine their exact number. This form of caregiving is not only relatively invisible, but the optimism prevalent in current medical research may also lead to the impression that most forms of pediatric disability are now preventable or curable. However, I believe that the numbers are growing and will likely continue to increase as medical advances at the borders of survival ensure an increasing number of effected children.

Extreme Dependency

Early theories within feminist ethics and an ethic of care were built on the observation that people are not, as other theories of ethics imply, fully competent and autonomous persons throughout our lives. In fact, all of us will be dependent on others at some point. We all required care during childhood and will likely require it again in sickness or old age. Eva Feder Kittay, in her analysis of caregiving presented in *Love's Labor* (1999), points out that there are fluctuating levels of dependency throughout our lives, beginning with the "utter dependency" of infancy through the relative independence of nondisabled adulthood (Kittay, 1999, p. 76). She states that some theories of care balance out the vulnerability and dependency incurred during those times, with the ability at other, more independent times to provide care to others. For example, a daughter might balance the care her mother gave her when she was a child by, in turn, caring for her mother in old age.

However, Kittay notes that there are some people, including Kittay's daughter Sesha, who remain in the dependent state of infancy or childhood outside those expected periods. Sesha has profound intellectual disabilities. Her development never progressed beyond infancy, and she remains profoundly dependent on others for almost every aspect of her daily living. Sesha and others like her are not able to return the care they have received or equalize their dependent status by performing care work for others. Kittay refers to this state as "extreme" dependency (p. xii), and discusses the implications of this extended state of vulnerability and dependency. People who are utterly dependent throughout their lives require a good deal of care (or dependency work) and cannot in turn balance the equation by providing care for others.

I propose that, if there are people who exhibit extreme dependency, it follows that they must require a similarly extreme level of caregiving. These extremely dependent people are exceptionally vulnerable to the actions of others and have no way to function as an equal in any contractual or autonomous arrangement. Nor can they be expected to provide a return on any utilitarian obligations to their caregiver. Their need is undeniable, however, and poses a moral obligation for care that falls upon the caregiver. They require, and the caregiver must provide, "extreme caregiving."

Kittay points out that caregiving for someone in total dependency can be morally demanding. She states, "Because the dependency worker is herself uniquely situated to harm or benefit her charge, the work itself carries a heavy moral load" (p. 49). In addition to doing the moral work of avoiding harm to her charge, the caregiver is herself vulnerable to domination or exploitation, particularly if she is situated as the only provider of desperate needs. The necessity to meet ongoing needs can cause the caregiver to give up more of herself (more time or energy) than she wishes or intends. In the face of overwhelming and undeniable need, the moral caregiver may not be able to disengage. This places the extreme caregiver in a uniquely vulnerable position. I agree with Kittay that support for the caregiver, or, as it is often stated in discussions of an ethic of care, "caring for the caregiver," is essential.

The need for extreme caregiving is not limited to people like Sesha who are totally dependent. While I do think Kittay has been and continues to be an example of an extreme caregiver for her daughter, I believe that there are situations of less dependency that also qualify as extreme. In the section on defining disability, I return to the variety of needs that might require parents to become extreme caregivers. It is important to note here that a close personal relationship, such as Kittay has with her daughter, is an important aspect of extreme caregiving. While Kittay extends her concepts of caring for someone in dependency to care workers outside of family, I largely talk about parents who are caring for their own children.

As parents, most of us expect to have to meet the needs of extreme dependency during the first few years of life. Infancy is indeed a situation of dependency. Parents are both uniquely positioned and usually able to meet the needs of their vulnerable infant. According to Kittay, this unique relationship calls forth a responsibility or a requirement to provide for needs, and parents are usually able to do so. She states, "We expect the parent to be willing to make the sacrifice" (p. 61). Kittay implies that this obligation to meet their own child's needs extends into the realm of total dependency, even if that dependency persists after infancy.

The term "special needs" has been used to describe children with any needs outside what is considered ordinary. This can include care during prolonged illnesses, the administration of complex medical home care, and support for a variety of physical and intellectual disabilities. Parents, then, become extreme caregivers because they are morally obligated to care for their child with needs outside the ordinary. These special needs, alone or in combination, often add up to caregiving that can be considered extreme.

Though professional caregivers, particularly in pediatrics, also provide care for children with special needs, I do not believe that professional caregiving often becomes extreme. Caregiving in a professional setting, such as pediatric hospitals, is usually done by nurses, who carry out the often unrecognized work of care. This work can be difficult, and often stressful, but it is compensated and constrained by training and employment conditions. Hospital health care workers are trained in the work of medical caregiving: to maintain IVs, give medications, change dressings, watch monitors, and connect gastric feeding tubes. Their job includes payment for some of the ordinary, messy tasks as well: diapers to be changed, baths to be given, and beds to be cleaned. But though the need is 24/7, health care workers, of course, have shifts. No matter how busy, at some point the work of caring can be passed to someone else.

It is when we shift to the home environment to provide this same level of care that I believe caregiving becomes extreme. The parents, essentially called upon to do all of the above, are placed in a new and uniquely difficult situation. They have not chosen medical caregiving as a career, they are not paid for their care work, nor are they fully trained in it. Yet, they must do all the work of nursing, while also continuing to maintain the home environment, including earning a living. They must be both parents and medical caregivers, round-the-clock and with no scheduled relief.

There is another aspect I believe is unique to extreme caregiving, which is the intimate relationship that already exists between parent and child. While relationships do develop between professional caregivers and patients, the care is usually being provided to someone who starts out as a stranger, with whom there are no past emotional ties or conflicts. Professional caregivers sometimes are called on to meet emotional needs as well as the physical needs of the child, but with parents that support is expected full time.

Parents of chronically ill children often have difficulty fulfilling the role of parent while also providing medical caregiving, particularly if that care requires performing unpleasant or painful procedures. It can also be difficult for a highly involved parent to leave the role of caregiver to others when necessary. Even when there are professional health care workers present, because of emotional ties, the parents' responsibilities cannot easily be left behind (Kirk, 1998). This emotional connection may be the most distinctive part of extreme caregiving, at once its most difficult and, possibly, most desirable aspect. Much of this book will center on an attempt to understand the impacts and evaluate the consequences of the emotional component of parent caregiving.

Extreme caregiving, then, involves the taking on of professional medical roles by a parent, who is not usually a trained medical caregiver, in a home environment. It can be complicated by medical complexity, and it often involves juggling multiple time-consuming tasks. The work must be carried out while maintaining a home or career (or both) and is usually done without respite. And, most importantly, extreme caregiving is performed for a person with whom the caregiver has an intense and personal relationship.

Parenting versus Extreme Caregiving

Within an ethic of care, caregiving is understood as necessary work, done to fulfill a need. Caregiving in a broader definition can include the meeting of any need, from feeding the hungry to cleaning the environment, but it is most often thought of as an individual meeting the needs of another. It can be done by either professionals or nonprofessionals. Parenting is certainly a form of nonprofessional caregiving and has its own unique problems and rewards.

Typical parenting has fairly well-defined parameters and expectations. Parents are expected to, at a bare minimum, keep the child fed, healthy, and safe from physical harm. But most agree that parenting also involves fostering independence and allowing the child to grow into a happy, free, and productive adult (Malek, 2009). There are certainly times when this is not an easy task. However, there are numerous sources of advice and support, and, when the child reaches adulthood, for better or worse, the dependency eventually ends.

Extreme caregiving includes these expectations of ordinary parenting. But the addition of meeting multiple medical needs causes an increase in the difficulty and complexity of care. Caring for an infant or toddler is more time-consuming than for an older child. Care of a child with an illness at any age is more difficult. Most parents can remember those sleepless nights when their child had a routine cold or fever. For children with special health care needs, ordinary nights are often sleepless and colds or fevers can be life-threatening. So a task that is already difficult is often punctuated by times when acute illness makes it even more demanding.

Lynne Ray, a nurse and researcher, in a 2002 paper based on interviews with thirty families of children with a variety of special needs, including medical fragility (frequent or severe medical problems, often triggered by minor illnesses) and technology dependence (need for medical equipment such as feeding tubes, monitors, and ventilators), identified a similar level of exceptional caregiving. The parents she interviewed were performing complex medical care, of the sort usually done only by specially trained hospital personnel. Some of the families in the study were providing home health care on a level that rivaled hospital or even pediatric ICU care (Ray, 2002). I outline the multiplicity of those tasks in more detail in later chapters.

Ray also recognized that many of the children in her study had severe delays in development and would, essentially, never outgrow their need for care. She called parenting these children, where stages of infancy and childhood can persist over an entire lifetime, "parenting plus." Some stay as dependent as infants throughout their lives. Others advance to toddlerhood, or even childhood, but still remain significantly dependent on others as adults. The prolongation of difficult stages of infancy or childhood, possibly throughout an entire life, is one of the most challenging aspects of extreme caregiving.

The care most of the children in Ray's study required was actually more difficult than parenting a typical infant or toddler, however. The parents were often also dealing with chronic illness, and on the front line of their child's medical care. They were responsible for "accurately diagnosing, and managing worrisome symptoms, complications, or emergencies" (Ray, 2002, p. 427). She describes a physically demanding, time-consuming, and emotionally difficult form of caregiving. Some "parenting plus" was being done in constant fear for their children's lives, magnifying both the emotional burden and the difficulty of fulfilling basic parental duties.

Not surprisingly, just as this combination of parenting and medical caregiving extends the parameters of parenting, it does not fall easily into understood forms of medical caregiving. Extreme caregiving often does involve a good deal of medical expertise, but it does not share the same goals as medical nursing. In a book promoting an ethic of medical care that is expanded to include palliation to ease dying, Joseph J. Fins provides a list of the goals of medical care: cure, restoring function, prolonging life, and comfort care/palliation (2006, p. 226). The sort of care that these parents are providing, while it might be informed by expectations promoted by these goals, is not really included in any of them. For many of these children, there is no overall cure available. Parents and physicians instead must pursue a variety of treatments and adaptations that will help the child. Instead of working to restore function that has been lost, they must engage in an ongoing pursuit of incremental improvements in abilities. Because these children are usually at the beginning of their lives, the concept of end-of-life care is not very useful. Likewise, while some children do require pain management, that palliation is rarely comfort care to ease dying. Extreme caregiving then confuses the expectations and goals of both typical parenting and medical caregiving.

For some, the parental duty to prevent physical harm must be redefined, particularly when a child's life depends on the parents performing painful medical procedures. Parents of ventilator-dependent children have reported difficulty performing the dual roles of parent and nurse when they were required to perform necessary but painful activities, particularly tracheal suctioning. The physical therapy needed to prevent contraction of spasmed muscles can also be uncomfortable for the child. Parents see their role during illness as comforting the child, and they found the need to do these uncomfortable procedures as stepping into a different role, which sometimes seemed in opposition to their expected role as parents (Kirk et al., 2005).

At times, even the definition of health needs to be reinterpreted. Savannah (the child we met in the Preface), who has multiple physical and intellectual disabilities, has been hospitalized for everything from congestive heart failure, to hip surgery, to feeding problems. For the first few years of her life, she could be fed only via a gastrostomy tube (GT), turning the fulfillment of a basic need into a medical procedure. Because of her complex problems, her individual definition of "healthy" had to take into account her GT feedings, multiple medications, and a heart monitor. There were times when, for her, being healthy meant merely not being in the hospital.

A final difference between the established goals of parenting and those of extreme caregiving comes as a direct result of delays in development. The prolonged dependency brought about by frequent illnesses, developmental disabilities, or intellectual delays complicates the parental duty of fostering independence. This can be as temporary as an interruption in school due to a hospitalization, or a much longer process, such as when adolescent separation from parents is delayed by the need for parents to monitor medical care. For some families of children with intellectual disabilities, however, the parameters of independence are fundamentally altered. At age eight, Savannah was walking but not talking or understanding, and essentially still needed to be cared for as though she was a toddler. By then it was becoming obvious that, as with many such intellectually delayed children, she would never reach a stage of self-sufficiency or independence.

Fostering independence in a child is one of the most important tasks of parenting. Parents must guide development, allowing the child the freedom to express himself while also keeping him safe from unwise choices and actions. Parents hold the child's identity as a person and must be careful not to force the child into a mold in which he does not fit. Joel Feinberg (1980) has proposed in addition that children have a right to what he calls an "open future." He asserts that parents are responsible for keeping open as many possibilities for their child's future as they can, so when the child reaches independent adulthood, there are no limitations on their life choices.

Parents also create a life story for the child who is not yet able to do it for himself. According to Hilde Lindemann (2014), as part of the process of adding new members, families construct stories that form a child's identity within the family. Some of these identities are obvious, like place of birth and number of siblings. Other identities are more precariously formed, often from preconceived parental expectations. These may need to be changed or rejected as the child grows in his ability to express his true self. Again, parents must be careful to hold the child's identity in a way that allows him freedom to take over and begin to tell his unique story as he enters adulthood.

Many of the children I have defined as requiring extreme care do not have the intellectual capability to ever reach the independence required for fully autonomous adulthood. Their futures are already limited, and their stories are already different from what the parents might have expected. The child's ability to express himself may also be limited. Children with severe delays, who may never be able to express anything beyond the most basic of needs will require prolonged assistance in the shaping and telling of their unique life story. That story must instead continue to be constructed, and their personhood defined, by their parents. The consequences of this are enormous and relatively unexplored, and this is the topic of the chapter on responsiveness.

This need to nurture a fragile personhood and sometimes limited autonomy is one of the things that separates extreme caregiving, not just from parenting, but also from other forms of caregiving. I am aware that caregiving at points in life other than childhood can be extreme in its difficulty and emotional demands. Spouses caring for their partner through serious illness will possibly be called upon to provide prolonged or specialized caregiving, as will the adult children of parents with dementia or who are dependent at the end of their lives. Extreme caregiving for children with multiple health care needs, I believe, is more challenging, because it requires the cultivation and sustenance of someone who has not yet had a chance, and might never be able, to declare themselves fully as their own person.

Defining Disability

Before we proceed to a discussion of the consequences of extreme caregiving, it is important to understand the range of illnesses or disabling conditions that parents must care for. There is, however, no specific medical category into which the children requiring extreme caregiving fall. Nor is there a precise definition of what counts as a "disabling condition" or an accepted way of discussing the severity of a disability.

I have said that the children who require extreme caregiving encompass a broad range of diagnoses, ages, and medical needs. Likewise they cross many of the boundaries of medicine and research. So while there are few studies specifically about them, there are many areas of study that indirectly involve them. They can be difficult to recognize within those studies, but they are there, at the most severe end of the spectrum of hundreds of illnesses. The largest and most studied of these groups is probably the survivors of neonatal intensive care units (NICU).

NICU survivors are often followed at a single center for long periods of time after discharge, and premature babies are a relatively homogeneous group, making them an ideal cohort to study. The vast neonatology literature on survivors of premature birth should be a source of information on the extent of disability and the consequences for the parent caregivers. There are, in fact, dozens of papers providing statistics for problems encountered in the NICU, at all levels of gestational age and situation at birth. Many additional studies contain outcome data, including types of disability, from years of follow-up after discharge.

Unfortunately, very few of these studies provide any kind of picture of the lives of their subjects. Part of the problem is that the need for caregiving has not been the focus of many studies, which tend instead to use established quality of life or mental health assessments. Additionally, there is a large discrepancy in the definition of disability used for each study, making it very difficult to examine the range of need that might be present in the study subjects.

In addition, the terminology of disability has changed drastically in the past few decades. The words used to diagnose and quantify levels of disability have evolved as medical knowledge has advanced, and as people with disabilities struggle to be recognized and celebrated in society. I am aware that the words used to describe disability, particularly intellectual disability, often become charged with negative meaning over time.

My brother's medical diagnosis, conferred upon him in the 1960s, was "trainable mentally retarded." This had a precise but rather inaccurate meaning at the time. We considered this a vast improvement over the prior terms "cretin" and "idiot," both of which had specific medical meaning in earlier decades. The word "retarded" is now similarly used as an insult. Nonetheless, we used it as a medical term so often when my brother was growing up that its current usage seems to me to have nothing to do with my brother. His story sometimes makes more sense in the language that was used at the time. The word retarded thus becomes both an accurate depiction of my brother's past and a reminder of how far we have come.

In the course of this book, I will be referring to sources, both researched studies and parent experiences, that span several decades. It is often not practical to translate the words of either researcher or parent into more modern usage. I will use whatever terminology the authors were most comfortable with in their writing, regardless of their current potentially inappropriate meanings. I apologize in advance for any offense this might cause.

My brother's level of "mental retardation" was diagnosed using a scale based on delayed developmental stages and an early version of an IQ test. At the time, many forms of developmental delay and intellectual disability, including autism, fell under this banner. "Mental retardation" was divided by IQ testing into "profound," "trainable," and "educable." My brother's years in what passed then for special education allowed me to make my own personal observations about what those words meant. The kids who were called "profound" did little except sit in their wheelchairs and moan. Most of them could not talk and were still in diapers in middle school. My brother was considered to be "trainable," and by middle school could do some of his own personal care. He was able to walk and talk, though his gait was unsteady and his words were slow and difficult to understand. Those kids who were "educable" were able to read a few words and do simple math. My brother's lifelong friend Karl, who had Down syndrome, was considered "educable." As an adult, he worked as a bagger at a nearby grocery store. He was never completely independent and lived with a full-time caregiver until his death at age fifty-eight, probably from a stroke. Today, neither the tests used to measure IQ nor the description of the results—"profound," "trainable," or "educable mental retardation"—is still in use. My interpretations are completely unscientific, based on my observations over time of a few of my brother's similarly diagnosed friends.

Current descriptions are more precise, but still, to my thinking, unhelpful without interpretation. The most complete summary of childhood disability in NICU survivors that I could find is a NICU follow-up study done in the UK in 2005. Neil Marlow's group followed a cohort of survivors of extremely premature birth (delivery before 26 weeks of gestation, or three to four months early) and conducted extensive developmental assessments when the children were six years old. I suspect, but of course cannot confirm, that the parents of every child in the study had been or continued to be extreme caregivers. The resulting paper is rife with statistical analyses based on complicated cognitive, neuromotor, and sensory evaluations, but it provides very little description of the actual level of functioning of their 241 subjects. The authors point out that there is a lack of a consistent definition of severe, moderate, or mild disability. They feel that their study is an improvement because of their precise definitions and measurements (Marlow et al., 2005). Their definitions are indeed the most comprehensive I was able to find.

Marlow's group defined the level of disability as severe if "it was considered likely to make the child highly dependent on caregivers and if it included nonambulant cerebral palsy, an IQ score more than 3 SD [standard deviations] below the mean, profound sensorineural hearing loss, or blindness" (p. 10). I translate this to mean that those children were confined to bed or a wheelchair, had extremely low IQs, or were blind or deaf. I suspect many had all of those problems. Likely some were unable to respond verbally, or suck from a bottle, or swallow food. "Highly dependent on caregivers" I believe means dependent on caregivers for every aspect of their daily existence. I will also be using the terms profound disability and total dependency to refer to the children in this group.

Marlow's group defined a disability as moderate if "reasonable independence was likely to be reached and if it included ambulant cerebral palsy, an IQ score 2 to 3 SD below the mean, sensorineural hearing loss that was corrected with a hearing aid, and impaired vision without blindness" (p. 11). Thus, for purposes of the study, "reasonable independence" consisted of being able to communicate somewhat and not be completely confined to bed or a wheelchair. They did not define "reasonable independence," but based on IQ scores, I suspect that Marlow's definition of moderate disability would include Savannah, who was able by age six to walk unassisted, communicate in limited sign language, and see a little bit if she held things close to her thick glasses. I would not expect someone who is that impaired at age six to develop the ability to live as a fully independent adult.

Mild disability included "neurologic signs with minimal functional consequences or other impairments such as squints or refractive errors" (p. 11). This group included those children with IQ scores from 1 to 2 SD below the mean. My brother, who has some spasticity but is able to walk and needed glasses only as he aged, would fall into this group. His Individual Service Plan states that he is "in the mild range of intellectual disability." (However, it also reports that his IQ is 54, which would place him in the profound category. There is no way to find out which test was used, when it was administered, or whether it was done correctly. This difficulty in categorizing a person who I know well demonstrates both the unreliability of IQ scoring and the problem with scoring the level of disability for anyone.) For him, developmentally, this meant saying his first words at age five, taking his first steps at age seven, and going to the toilet by himself at around age ten. At age fifty, he was not able to live independently. Some of these kids, those with IQs in the 70s, might eventually reach full independence, but would, I suspect, require quite a lot of assistance to achieve it.

Neither the system used to diagnose my brother, nor Marlow's more extensive measurements, consider the implications for current or future caregiving needs. The level of care required was not measured, nor was there any discussion of the effects of the disability on the child or family. The lack of this information makes classifying levels of caregiving impossible. It is obvious that caregiving becomes more difficult as disability becomes more profound, but there is no way to correlate either diagnosis or level of impairment with difficulty in caregiving. For this reason, I will make no attempt to establish a cut-off where caregiving becomes extreme. It is pointless to argue over who is, and is not, providing extreme care.

However, I must clarify the widely disparate problems that are united by the complexity and ongoing nature of "special needs." There are several categories of need that I believe are likely to require extreme caregiving. They are complex medical needs, physical disability, intellectual disability, and communication problems. All of these have, of course, degrees of severity, with the need for extreme caregiving falling only at the worst-affected end of a spectrum. Many children fall into several categories.

"Complex medical needs" encompasses children with chronic medical problems requiring multiple medications and doctor visits. Some of these children are dependent on home medical technology, such as home ventilators, tube feedings, and monitors. Others have numerous medical problems involving multiple bodily systems, and so require multiple pediatric specialists and numerous medications. Often, this form of need decreases with time, as some problems stabilize or improve with growth. I have not included in this category children with a single chronic disease, such as asthma, or severe but often temporary illnesses, such as childhood cancer. I believe that these parents must indeed perform extreme caregiving, at least for a time, but the long-term consequences are likely quite different, and I did not include memoirs of such parenting in my study.

Isolated physical impairments such as blindness, deafness, epilepsy, and physical disabilities also do not necessarily lead to a need for extreme caregiving, though some of the consequences and emotional adaptations that parents need to make in the face of disability are similar. However there are constellations of problems, such as spina bifida and severe cerebral palsy, that do require prolonged or lifetime assistance. In addition, many of these impairments are found in conjunction with other problems that result in extreme dependency. Mild to moderate impairments of vision, hearing, and mobility, in combination with intellectual delays, a common circumstance, increases and prolongs the level of dependency.

Intellectual disability is probably the easiest scale on which to predict the need for extreme caregiving. Mild disabilities, such as learning disabilities or behavior problems, are not easy for parents and child but unlikely in isolation to engender severe dependency. However, moderate to severe levels of intellectual disability result in a delay in development that can prolong childhood stages or delay the attainment of independence. These children do continue to attain new skills as they grow, so their care can become easier over time. But even the least impaired of children with intellectual disability, who are often referred to as "high functioning," are likely to require some assistance into adulthood.

Profound intellectual disability is very rarely found in isolation. I will use the terms severe and profound synonymously, and only to refer to children and adults with global dependency. These children are totally dependent for their entire lives. They often cannot suck or swallow well, and so require tube or slow bottle feedings. If they are unable to move independently, their need for care increases as they grow up, as feeding and performing personal hygiene tasks become more difficult. Their care, in my estimation, defines the hardest of extreme caregiving.

The final category I have included is communication problems. While this is indeed a part of other types of disability, such as intellectual delay or deafness, including it as a separate category here allows me to include memoirs from parents of children with autism in my study. Many of the issues that arise in severe autism are very similar to those that arise with moderate to severe intellectual disability. In many children with autism, difficulty in communication alone can result in prolonged dependency. For many, communication skills improve with time and care becomes easier. However, if a child with autism (or intellectual disability) continues to be unable to communicate verbally, severe behavior problems can result from misunderstanding directions or frustration at being unable to express needs. As the child reaches the teenage years, behavior outbursts backed by increasing size can have devastating results, vastly increasing the difficulty of giving care.

I want to stress again that the pathways to extreme caregiving are many and varied, and most have not previously been considered to be related. They encompass common diagnoses such as autism and Down syndrome, along with many obscure syndromes, like Cornelia DeLang syndrome or Trisomy 18. Disability can arise from premature birth, genetic diseases, inborn physical anomalies, and severe accidents or illness. The children have a combination of fragile health, multiple physical disabilities, mild to profound intellectual disabilities, and communication problems. Many have all of those at once. They have in common a need for prolonged and intense care, usually provided by their parents.

Quantifying Extreme Caregiving

Because of the multiple and varied conditions that can lead to disabilities that require children to be cared for at home by nonprofessionals, we cannot accurately count the number of children requiring complex care at home. Despite this, we need to recognize that they are a significant and growing group. Extreme caregiving exists across a spectrum of pediatric diseases and conditions, at the most severe end of hundreds of syndromes. While physicians, researchers, and scholars study many of these children as representatives of their various problems, they do not often address their common need for increased care. Those who stand at a remove from extreme caregiving, or to whom caregiving is invisible, do not think of the children in question as a group united by their need for care. In part as a result of this, many do not grasp the intensity of the caregiving they require or see the scope or scale of this phenomenon.

Most statistics available for medically complex children are gathered within fairly narrow parameters. Papers in the medical literature might estimate, for example, the number of children with one specific diagnosis, but statistics for the number of children suffering from a single syndrome will include a range of levels of severity. They usually do not attempt to number the sickest children whose care would be expected to be the most intense, nor do they usually include an evaluation of the extent of home care required for any of the children on that disease spectrum.

There are some statistics on the number of children who are dependent specifically on the use of medical technology in the home. Technology dependence is, I believe, a fairly good marker for a high level of home care, though again the range of illnesses and severity is enormous. Susan Kirk, writing in 1998 on technology-dependent children in Britain, reported that the number of technology-dependent children in the United States ten years earlier, in 1988, was estimated to be around 100,000, and increasing at a rapid pace. The types of technology available included mechanical ventilation, home oxygen, home IV therapy, peritoneal dialysis, and tube feedings (Kirk, 1998). Of course, this number measures only those children who require medical technology at home and does not include the number of children whose lack of need for advanced equipment in no way lowers their need for care.

Another source of data, though also almost twenty years out of date, is a 1998 study done by the Minnesota Department of Health, Division of Family Health (MDHDFH), surveying families on Minnesota's TEFRA program. TEFRA is Minnesota's program for financial assistance to families with disabled children who require excess expensive medical care. (The acronym stands for Tax Equity Fairness and Responsibility Act, the law which established the criteria for the program. No one uses the full name, and the word TEFRA is commonly used to refer to every part of the implementation of the Act, from the forms filled out to the payments received.) To qualify for this assistance, children must be "disabled with a physical or mental impairment that is comparable in severity to one that would prevent an adult from working and that is expected to last at least 12 months, or results in death." An additional eligibility requirement is that the children must need "the level of care provided in a hospital, nursing home or Intermediate Care Facility for Persons with Mental Retardation" (Chan et al., 1998, p. 13).

In 1995, the MDHDFH funded a study to determine characteristics of the children and families benefiting from TEFRA. Questionnaires were sent to half of the families of the 3,770 children enrolled, and 959 of them responded. Diagnoses ranged from spina bifida to autism, from cancer to mental retardation, with many children carrying multiple diagnoses (Chan et al., 1998, p. 24). The type of care these children required depended, of course, on their specific diagnosis and was often very different. The level of care and the time consumed in the giving of that care was not directly measured, but 82% of the parents reported that their children required constant or frequent supervision, and "about one-fifth" of the parents reported that their children were "totally dependent in all activities of daily living" (p. 2). From this, we can extrapolate that almost all of the nearly 4000 children on TEFRA required extreme caregiving, with about 20% of them requiring assistance with every aspect of their daily lives. Interestingly, part of the reason the survey was done was to document that the families receiving assistance were truly in need of the enormous level of financial outlay incurred by the program.

It is not unreasonable to assume that the population of Minnesota is representative of the rest of the United States and that the proportion of extreme caregivers is no different in the other forty-nine states. According to 2010 census data provided by Wikipedia, Minnesota holds about 2% of the population of the United States. Multiplying the 4000 children on TEFRA, we can presume that there are about 200,000 children nationwide. This is likely an underestimation, since not every child who requires extreme care in Minnesota is on TEFRA, which is given mostly to families on medical assistance or with limited insurance and is provided, in part, on a financial need basis. Nor does TEFRA extend past childhood, which, as we have seen, is not a limitation on extreme caregiving. It is also based on a figure from 1995, which has almost certainly increased since then. I would guess the number by now has at least doubled.

This guess is borne out in a more recent estimate of numbers of children requiring extreme caregiving, which comes from Andrew Solomon's 2012 book, *Far From the Tree*. Solomon's seventh chapter discusses parents coping with children with multiple severe disability, or MSD. He defines MSD as considerable impairment in several areas of sensory ability or cognition, and he states that it refers to people with an "overwhelming number of challenges," many of which will never resolve enough to permit independent living. He reports, "Although the vagueness of the criteria for MSD makes it much harder to collate the relevant statistics than it is for single, clearly defined conditions, about twenty thousand children with MSD are born in the United States each year" (Solomon, 2012, p. 357). He also states that it has only been in the last twenty years that parents have been expected to bring home and care for such children. This estimate would indicate that there are somewhere around 400,000 families doing extreme caregiving, doubling my TEFRA-based estimate. This would include only children with MSD under twenty years old.

These numbers do not include another source of the need for extreme caregiving, which is autism. The results of studies done by the Center for Disease Control and Prevention (CDC) on autism spectrum disorder (ASD) have been highly publicized, as have the data that diagnoses of ASD have been climbing rapidly. The most recent study, reported in April of 2016 states that the incidence is one in sixty-eight (CDC, 2016). This says very little about the severity of problems over the entire spectrum of the condition, however. The total number of people living with severe autism has not been reliably estimated, nor has the percentage of children with autism who require extreme caregiving. I think it is safe to assume that tens of thousands of families, at least, are providing care for children and adults at the most severe end of the autism spectrum.

In 2009 and 2010, the CDC conducted a nationwide survey of households with children, looking specifically for the number of children with special health care needs (CSHCN). Their definition of CSHCN was quite broad and did include autism. It also included several diagnoses that do not often lead to a need for extreme caregiving, such as ADD/ADHD, asthma, depression, and migraines. About half of CSHCN were receiving family-provided home health care, for a total number of 5.5 million, however most of those were averaging only about five hours a week performing health care for their child. A subset of 11.7% of those families were likely doing extreme caregiving, reporting that they were providing over twenty-one hours a week of care (Romley et al., 2017). That would make the total estimate of children requiring extreme care somewhere around 650,000.

Another unknown is the number of elderly parents still caring for dependent adult sons and daughters. This is an unexplored aspect of caregiving, a very prolonged form of parenting combined with medical caregiving that falls in the parameters of extreme caregiving. As with the population of parents doing extreme caregiving for younger children, there is no complete or accurate count. A 2001 estimate of mentally retarded, developmentally disabled, or intellectually disabled adults placed their numbers at about 3.24 million. Of these, about 60% (about 1.94 million) were still living with their parents, however the actual level of disability and need for care was not reported (Braddock et al., 2001).

An estimate of about 600,000 children under the age of twenty in the United States living at home with some combination of multiple severe disability, severe autism, or technology dependence would not be unrealistic. There may be an additional million or so adults with similar disabilities who are still depending on their parents for care. This places the total number of families who are doing this sort of extreme caregiving at somewhere around one-and-a-half million. I believe the actual number is much higher.

Trending Statistics

Without accurate statistics it is also not possible to pinpoint a trend in the number of children requiring complex care. Based on Solomon's (2012) assertion that 20,000 children with MSD are born each year, it follows that there has been a steady increase in both number of children and in the complexity of their care. This would lead to a conclusion that, despite advances in pediatrics, particularly in neonatology, there is an apparent increase in MSD in children.

We have come to depend on medical science for a constant stream of improvements: new medications, more effective treatments, and increased life expectancy. This has not, however, led to a decreased need for caregiving. In fact, the prolongation of life in old age, for example, has led to a seeming crisis, as an expanding older population seeks the care they need. Likewise, medical advances in pediatrics have seemingly contributed to an increase in the need for parental caregiving. We should understand why advancing science is increasing, rather than decreasing or eliminating, the number of children who require extreme caregiving.

It is true that there has been amazing progress in neonatology. When my brother was born in 1960, the second of twins delivered two months early, at 32 weeks, he was at a significant disadvantage to a baby born at the same gestational age today. A child born at 32 weeks today would have the benefit of accurately adjustable oxygen administration; the ability to constantly monitor blood oxygen levels; miniscule IVs to ensure adequate hydration; and tiny, flexible tubes that pass easily from nose to stomach to provide nutrition. My mother also would have been monitored constantly during delivery and would have had a C-section at the first sign of distress. These few improvements would have almost certainly prevented the most likely source of my brother's brain damage, which was probably due to lack of oxygen during and after delivery. It is possible that what happened to my brother was a prenatal stroke, which even today is not preventable, but for every other possibility, born today, my brother would not be intellectually disabled.

In 1960, a baby born at 28 weeks (three months early) could rarely be saved, but by 1990, just as the statistics for 32 weeks began to improve, those same advances made it possible for the survival of 28-week preemies to become routine. Of course, many of the survivors of 28-week pregnancies were mildly to severely disabled. Today, though birth at 28 weeks is still a difficult beginning, the long-term outcome is much better. But advances have not stopped. It is now possible to save babies born even earlier, at 23 to 25 weeks, a full four months early. Delivery at 25 weeks was, in 1960, called miscarriage. It still is in much of the world today. At this writing, it is still legal in most of the United States to have an abortion through 24 weeks. But resuscitation of 23- to 25-week preemies in high-level NICUs is becoming fairly routine, though survival is precarious. The survival rates at 24 and 25 weeks seem to be slowly improving but still hover around 50%. Survival at 23 weeks, however, remains steady at a bit less than 20%, and survival at 22 weeks hovers around zero (Field et al., 2008).

There is a high level of disability in those survivors. A recent study of surviving 23-to 25-week preemies found that only 20% of their subjects could be described as having no disability. At six years of age, about one-fifth (22%) of the survivors were found to be "severely" disabled, about one-quarter (24%) "moderately" disabled, and about one-third (34%) "mildly" disabled (Marlow et al., 2005). We have seen that the terms "severe," "moderate," or "mild" disability all correspond to an expectation of a high need for caregiving. Even those children with no disability apparent at age six would have been in the NICU for months, and likely required at least a few months of extreme caregiving after discharge from the hospital.

Of course, further advancement in neonatology will undoubtedly provide better outcomes for future infants born before 26 weeks. Just as advancement in the care of ever-smaller preemies resulted in surer outcomes for the 28- to 32-weekers, it can be expected that survival and outcome for the micro-preemie will improve. If, at the same time, the boundary for survival is pushed even lower, to 22 weeks or less, the overall number of ex-preemies surviving with disabilities is unlikely to decrease.

Boundaries are being pushed in other neonatal areas as well. Trisomy 18 is a genetic syndrome involving multiple abnormalities including severe deformities of the heart and brain. In medical school in the 1970s, I was taught very little about it, because it was very rare, and felt to be uniformly fatal. The *Harriet Lane Handbook*, which I carried with me for years as my pediatric guidebook, stated, up through its 2002 edition, that all but 10% of these babies died in their first year, and all had "profound mental retardation" (Gunn & Nechyba, 2002, p. 330). As late as 2006, the recommendation was to cease resuscitation as soon as the diagnosis was confirmed by genetic testing. By 2014, however, a survey of neonatologists at high-level NICUs in New York found that very few neonatologists would not at least consider resuscitation, even if the infant had severe anomalies such as a complex congenital heart condition requiring open-heart surgery (McGraw & Perlman, 2008). With ongoing resuscitation, ventilation, and multiple surgeries, a neonatology center in Japan has raised the survival rate at one year to 25% (Kosho et al., 2006). Some of these infants have been discharged from the NICU and have been able to go home. This raises the possibility that survival might continue to improve and that the cessation of resuscitation due to the expectation of fatality is a self-fulfilling prophecy. All of those children are profoundly intellectually disabled, however, and certainly require extreme caregiving.

I find it interesting that, at the same time as resuscitation is being recommended for ever-more precarious infants, widespread genetic testing has become available to screen for similar problems. It is not my intent here to discuss the appropriateness (and also the discordance) of this. But I must mention the likely effect of prenatal testing on the population of a more common and much less severe trisomy, Trisomy 21, better known as Down syndrome. According to a study from the UK, although termination rates after the confirmation of a fetus with Down syndrome remain steady at approximately 92%, the overall birthrate of Down syndrome infants has fallen only by 1%. The authors attribute this to an increase in average maternal age, which would have led to a large increase in the number of babies born with Down syndrome, if not offset by the termination rate (Morris & Alberman, 2009). A study done in the United States shows that the termination rate is seemingly falling, to around 67 to 85%, depending on the population studied. Younger women, particularly, have not chosen termination, perhaps due to changes in societal attitudes toward disability. The author reports that the decrease may be due to "progress in medical management . . . and advances in educational, social, and financial support" (Natoli et al., 2012). Considering the two factors—increasing maternal age and the emergence of selective genetics—there has been perhaps a small decrease in the number of Down syndrome births in the United States (Egan et al., 2004), though the prevalence of Down syndrome births worldwide seems to have remained stable (Cocchi et al., 2010).

An expectation that genetic screening for Trisomy 21 and other genetic problems will result in the birth of fewer children with disabilities is widespread. The very slight decrease in births of children with Down syndrome hints that this will not be a successful endeavor, however. Not only are there significant ethical questions raised by this form of genetic selection, but also such screening will never be able to eliminate all forms of genetic differences. Nor is there agreement on which, if any, disabling conditions should be eliminated. In addition, many potentially disabling genetic combinations are not predictable or attributed to easily detectable genetic causes. We cannot expect medical science to prevent the need for extreme caregiving by this form of screening.

Another false expectation is that medical research will very soon decrease the number of children with disabilities by offering a variety of new cures and treatments. I am aware that many parents of children with disabilities reject the emphasis on cures, in part because the need for a cure implies that there is something terribly wrong with their children (Berube, 2016). But an uncounted number of parent organizations also fund drives for research into specific diagnoses, placing a great deal of hope in the possibility of a cure. No matter which discourse prevails, most of the presumed cures are very far off, and the number of affected children will likely remain unchanged.

If there are indeed concerns about parents becoming extreme caregivers, we cannot then stand aside and expect medical progress to provide solutions for us. In fact, if we continue to push the boundaries of medicine, as we must, I can anticipate no decrease in the number of children who require extreme care. I expect that the number is rising and will continue to rise, even as, and, in some cases *because*, advances on all medical fronts are being made.

While we have been distracted by medical progress, children have been born with, or are developing, disabilities that cause them to require a great deal of support to survive and thrive. The caregiving that their parents are providing for them is almost invisible next to the wonders of science which may have contributed to their survival. It is time to notice and support their efforts, and to understand the process of extreme caregiving. If these parents, as Kingsley suggests in her essay "Welcome to Holland," have had their lives rerouted to somewhere unexpected and, perhaps, alien, it is time to begin to map the place in which they landed.

With an estimated one-and-a-half million families doing the complex task that I have called extreme caregiving, defining the landscape of their task is not a trivial undertaking. We have seen that the children who require extreme caregiving are affected by a multitude of medical problems or disabling conditions. They also occupy a range from mild impairments requiring a lot of extra help, through profound compromise that can result in complete, lifelong dependence. No single area of medical research or endeavor encompasses them all. This book only begins to tell their stories and attempts to find both common ground and common concerns in caring for them.

Extreme caregiving falls randomly on families, when severe illness devastates a well child or, more often, when congenital problems result in a medically fragile or disabled infant. Extreme caregiving happens when a preemie is finally sent home from the NICU with a tracheostomy, feeding tube, home oxygen, apnea monitor, and a dozen or so different medications. It happens when an eight-year-old with Down syndrome remains developmentally in the active but clueless eighteen-month-old stage and has to be watched every second for years so he doesn't injure himself. It happens when a fourteen-year-old, 160-pound child with autism has not yet learned to use a toilet or sit at a table, and whose behavior outbursts, backed by increasing strength, are becoming destructive. The worrisome addition to these situations is that in ten years, or twenty, the level of care may be unchanged. Extreme caregiving also happens when a fifty-year-old, moderately intellectually delayed man, who is still functionally a five-year-old, remains in the care of his seventy-year-old mother whose own health is failing.

The task now is to find academic and medical studies that include families who are doing extreme caregiving and uncover the places where any problems discovered overlap with concerns expressed by those families in narrative. We will find numerous similarities in the seemingly disparate situations that I believe are united by the term extreme caregiving.

I hope by exploring this area to begin to provide a conceptual framework that can be extended to other care situations and used to elucidate the nature of caregiving itself. These parents are at the forefront of an ongoing revolution in home care, doing the most difficult of caregiving work, invisibly and without recognition. If the medical system continues to promote ever-more-difficult levels of home care, we must understand the practical reality of the lives these parents lead. We must understand why families agree to take on the new burden of care, and how they arrange their lives around it. We must acknowledge the physical and emotional burden imposed by complex and prolonged caregiving. But mostly we must understand the intense relationship that forms between a parent, who is also the provider of medical care, and a child who is the recipient of such superhuman, extreme caregiving.

CHAPTER 3 | Hard Labor

NOW THAT WE have established that quite a few parents are being called upon to do the task that I have called extreme caregiving, we need to review information that is already known about it. I have said that some pediatric literature hints at the existence of extreme caregiving, mostly in studies of pediatric home health care, psychological evaluations of parents of sick children, and investigations of quality of life in neonatal follow-up studies. There is also information to be found in the ethics literature, particularly in the scholarly nursing journals, where there are several interview-based ethical analyses of the problems encountered by families caring for technology-dependent children. The disability studies, anthropology, sociology, and feminist literature also touch on areas of extreme caregiving. All of these sources begin to illuminate some of the problems that arise in extreme caregiving.

Studies from the medical and ethical literature that shed some light on the lives of extreme caregivers are based mostly on interviews with the families of children with chronic complex medical problems. Many were conducted in countries other than the United States; they come from health care centers in the United Kingdom, Canada, and Norway. They largely present data from interviews with a small number of families with children who are dependent on a variety of types of home medical equipment, and so the studies cross a variety of syndromes and diagnoses (Kirk, 1998; Ray, 2002; Wang & Bernard, 2004; Kirk et al., 2005; Cockett, 2012). Some of the studies concern only families of children who are ventilator dependent, but even these represent multiple types of need (Carnevale et al., 2006; Dybwik et al., 2011). Based on the criteria for inclusion of families in all the studies, I have no doubt that all the parents interviewed were engaging in extreme caregiving. Because these studies also sometimes report direct quotes from parents, they are a source, not only of data, but of caregiving stories. The ways in which the stories are similar, despite disparate diagnoses, is intriguing.

The studies from the disability, sociology, and anthropology literature are mostly based on written or phone surveys (Green, 2003; Green, 2006; Trute et al., 2010; Lalvani, 2011). This method can reach a larger number of families, but the information acquired is not as detailed. It is possible that some of the parents involved in these surveys were not extreme caregivers, however, again based on inclusion criteria, I believe that most of them were. I also found several relevant essays and studies in the recent feminist literature on motherhood and disability (Layne, 1999; Landsman, 1999, Zebricky, 2014). These were mostly based on personal essays or extensive interviews, and left no doubt that the mothers who participated were extreme caregivers.

To achieve a more sophisticated and multidimensional understanding of extreme caregiving, we must correlate the scant information on caregiving from the academic literature with parents' testimony. In what follows I draw from personal experience, both as a sibling to an intellectually disabled brother and as a medical provider for a variety of children with special health care needs in my pediatric practice. But my largest source of narrative information was from parents' stories, published in memoirs and autobiographical essays.

As I was gathering information on the lived experience of parents of children with special needs, I came across various sources online. There are parent narratives on the websites of support groups, hospital-based "caring bridge" sites where parents report the ongoing experience of their child's illness, and numerous personal blogs. These were intriguing but less than satisfactory. With a few exceptions, the stories are told in brief, emotional paragraphs, with little connection or follow-up. Often they are written in the moment of crisis to inform friends and relatives about events or respond to a recent problem. In many of these forums, the narrators do not have to identify themselves. Of course, these parents were writing oftentimes to relieve pressure and exchange informal advice, not to serve as an academic's resource later on.[1]

It seemed best to rely on narratives published in print, preferably in a longer form. While this does give a chance for the author to craft a story,

---

[1] I have recently encountered numerous sources, mostly blog sites, that do contain reflective, analytic essays. Examples are David Parry's "How Did We Get Into This Mess? (www.thismess.net) and Laura MacGregor's "Love and Chaos" (www.extremecaregiving.com). There is indeed relevant information in sources like these, but finding and analyzing them is work for another time.

perhaps altering it for purposes of his own, at least there is a reflective process required in the months it takes to put that many words on paper. Rather than rely on fiction, which would be filtered through characters, I looked for first-person narratives written by parents of children with multiple disabilities or severe autism.

I also encountered narratives by people who grew up with disabilities. Certainly memoirs such as Lucy Grealy's *Autobiography of a Face* (1994) and Martin Pistorious's *Ghost Boy* (2013) have important things to tell us about being cared for. However, they rarely include the perspective of the caregiver. Several memoirs have also been written by siblings of disabled children.[2] But while siblings can, and do, participate in the caregiving process, as I know from my childhood with my intellectually disabled brother, I think it best, at this early stage, to focus only on the parents. In recounting experiences with my brother, I attempt to relate my parents' stories and draw from my own only in the final chapters. I am not sure whether my experience as a sibling makes me uniquely qualified for, or disqualifies me from, academic study of this topic.

My search for narratives was by necessity somewhat haphazard. I had to rely on word of mouth, internet listings of books recommended by various parent support groups, and searches of the shelves of libraries and book stores. There are not many parents who have so far shared their stories of living with the sort of disability that makes a parent into an extreme caregiver. My suspicion is that people doing the most difficult caregiving work do not have time to write memoirs. This is borne out by my finding that many, though certainly not all, of these narratives were written by fathers who had offices away from home, while their wives performed most of the care. More were written by parents, both mothers and fathers, after their caregiving task ended with either the death of the child or placement in a group home. They were also largely written by people who were writers before they became the parents of a disabled child. This may give them a slightly different perspective, yet it also gives them a unique and authentic voice.

Since caring is traditionally women's work, the largest burden of care often falls upon women and, as such, is relatively undervalued and underpaid (Noddings, 1994). This was not a theme of any of the research on technology-dependent children, where both fathers and mothers were interviewed (though there were more mothers than fathers), and the

---

[2] I recommend Karl Taro Greenfeld's *Boy Alone* (2000) and Rachel Simon's *Riding the Bus with My Sister* (2002), both of which provide insight into the lives of siblings of people with intellectual disabilities.

studies were too small to attempt separate analysis by gender. A review of the literature does mention that mothers were more likely than fathers to give up their jobs (Cockett, 2012), and there is an underlying assumption that mothers are doing most of the caregiving. However, I did not pursue more information on the gendered nature of extreme caregiving nor try to explore the reasons why many of the longer narratives I found were written by fathers.

I also did not explore the ways in which class or race might affect extreme caregiving. Most of the pediatric and ethics studies either did not mention their study demographics or did not obtain enough information from diverse populations to come to any conclusions. Several studies done in other English-speaking countries were available, but again there was not enough information to pinpoint any differences. I am also aware that all the parent narrators are white and that most of them are college educated. Therefore, much of the information on extreme caregiving obtained from these sources may not apply to diverse populations, particularly cultures where there are fewer resources or there are different views on the meaning of motherhood or disability.

The issues described in the disparate sources, while sometimes labeled differently, were remarkably similar. I chose a set of common themes from a list of concerns raised by the academic literature, particularly those which reviewed ethical concerns regarding caregiving for children with complex medical problems. All of these themes were frequently reflected in autobiographies written by parents of children with special needs. The similarities existed despite the fact that the researchers relied on families of technology-dependent children and the narrators were caring for children who were not, for the most part, dependent on any technology.

In this chapter I intend to correlate these disparate sources of information, both to begin to explore the difficulties encountered and to show that some of the stories told by parents are not exaggerated. I will begin with three of the most visible and easily documented aspects of extreme caregiving: the physical burdens, the financial difficulties, and the social consequences. I will then discuss the ways in which our cultural preference for positivity effectively silences parents who speak out about the hardships they encounter. I conclude with an example of opposing narratives of disability and how they play out in research on the quality of life of children with disabilities, as parents attempt to hold their child's place in a demanding world. Extreme caregiving is hard, expensive, and sometimes lonely work, and those who complain about it are often not appreciated.

The Physical Burden of Care

Walker Brown was born in 1996, and began having medical problems almost right away. He refused feedings, vomited often, cried all the time, and was frequently ill. By eight months his very astute pediatrician had diagnosed his particular set of illnesses, together with his somewhat unusual appearance, rough skin, and developmental delay, as a rare syndrome called CFC (Cardiofaciocutaneous syndrome). The diagnosis provided very little reassurance or certainty for his family, however. A syndrome is merely a collection of anomalies, allowing children with similar sets of problems to be grouped together. In this exceedingly rare syndrome, with known cases numbering only in the few hundreds, each child remains a special case. Though there are treatments for some of the problems that arise, there is no overall cure. There is not even enough knowledge to accurately predict individual long-term outcome.

By eight years of age, most of Walker's medical problems had stabilized, but his developmental delay was more obvious. He would not talk and showed no understanding when he was spoken to. He still refused to eat most solid foods, and so was fed at night by a continuous drip of formula through a gastrostomy tube into his stomach. He was, however, physically active, walking and running, and often successful at hurting himself. Of course, he could not feed himself, nor was he toilet trained. He woke every night, and had to be held tightly to prevent self-injurious behavior. Though tube feedings are probably the least complex of the medical technology available for home use, there is no question that Walker required extreme caregiving.

Walker's father, Ian Brown, described his life with Walker in a 2011 book called *The Boy in the Moon: A Father's Journey to Understand His Extraordinary Son*, which I think should be required reading for all who work in pediatric hospitals. The book opens with a vivid description of caring for Walker at age eight years. In the opening chapter, Brown's description of a typical night speaks volumes about the cost of continuous night feedings, this seemingly simple procedure.

> For the first eight years of Walker's life, every night is the same. The same routine of tiny details, connected in precise order, each mundane, each crucial . . .
>
> Tonight I wake up in the dark to a steady, motorized noise . . . *Nnngah.* Pause. *Nnngah. Nnngah* . . . It's my boy, Walker, grunting as he punches himself in the head, again and again . . .

> I count the grunts as I pad my way into his room: one a second. To get him to stop hitting himself, I have to lure him back to sleep, which means taking him downstairs and making him a bottle and bringing him back into bed with me.
>
> That sounds simple enough, doesn't it? But with Walker, everything is complicated. Because of his syndrome, he can't eat solid food by mouth or swallow easily. Because he can't eat, he takes in formula through the night via a feeding system. The formula runs along a line from a feedbag and a pump on a metal IV stand, through a hole in Walker's sleeper and into a clever-looking permanent valve in his belly, sometimes known as a G-tube, or mickey. To take him out of bed and down into the kitchen to prepare the bottle that will ease him back to sleep, I have to disconnect the line from the mickey. To do this, I first have to turn off the pump (in the dark, so he doesn't wake up completely) and close the feed line. If I don't clamp the line, the sticky formula pours out onto the bed or the floor (the carpet in Walker's room is pale blue: there are patches that feel like the Gobi Desert under my feet, from all the times I have forgotten). To crimp the tube, I thumb a tiny red plastic roller down a slide. (It's my favourite part of the routine—one thing, at least, is easy, under my control.) I unzip his one-piece sleeper, reach inside to unlock the line from the mickey, pull the line out through the hole in his sleeper and hang it on the IV rack that holds the pump and feedbag. Close the mickey, rezip the sleeper. Then I reach in and lift all 45 pounds of Walker from the depths of the crib. He still sleeps in a crib. It's the only way we can keep him in bed at night. He can do a lot of damage on his own. (Brown, 2011, pp. 1–2)

This is only a small part of the nighttime ritual, which takes another several pages to describe. It ends with Brown getting into bed with Walker and holding him through the rest of the night to keep him from hitting himself. Brown and his wife have been doing this every night, taking turns, neither of them ever really getting a full night's sleep, for eight years. The individual caregiving tasks that must be done, like the disconnection of the gastrostomy tube, are simple, but they are not always done in ideal conditions. The need to perform each task in exact sequence, together with the need to deal with the consequences of any mishaps, add up to an enormous amount of caregiving work.

The caregiving task given to Brown and other parents of children with special needs includes the work of parenting, such as feeding and diapering, as well as the work of nursing; giving medications, monitoring for illness, and, for some, maintaining technology. All parents know how time-consuming it is to care for a newborn who cannot do anything for himself, and for a toddler who not only still needs lots of help with ordinary things but also persists in getting into trouble. Clearly, adding a problem such as chronic or complex illness, technology dependence, or intellectual disability, is likely to compound that work. However, we are not in the habit of thinking about the small details of day-to-day existence and calculating the enormous volume of effort they might entail.

The caregiving work necessary to maintain a home and family has been devalued as "women's work" and has become (or, perhaps, has always been) somewhat invisible. Hands-on caregiving in the medical system, the always-present need for bringing comfort and cleaning up, is done by the lowest paid and often least valued medical workers (Noddings, 1984). The new computerized medical record systems, which exist in part to assure that no cost goes unnoticed and unpaid, usually do not bother to account for this important work, presumably because those who invented the systems did not recognize its existence or necessity. The caregiving that happens at home is even less visible and is often completely outside the concern and thoughts of medical providers. The people doing this work are themselves often unable to account for what they are doing. One family of a technology-dependent child reported that they "were so busy doing things for their child that they did not have time to think about" the extent of the work they were doing (Ray, 2002, p. 432). All of these factors contribute to the lack of a coherent account of the caregiving work that is being done.

Much of the available information on the nature and burden of the caregiving required by children with special needs has been obtained by interviewing parents of technology-dependent children who must be under frequent observation by medical providers. This can include a range of technology, from home IV therapy or gastrostomy feedings, to home dialysis or ventilator support. The reports are found mostly in the nursing literature. Though the children vary in diagnosis, age, and disability, the work parents are doing and the concerns they express are remarkably similar.

An early review of the families of technology-dependent children stated, "sleep deprivation due to anxiety about the child's condition, false monitor alarms or the need to remain vigilant over their child during the night" is a consistent theme (Kirk, 1998, p. 106). Others also report a high amount of sleeplessness and sleep deprivation, as well as "physical overburden" causing parental burnout and exhaustion even if the child's health is stable (Wang & Bernard, 2004). Ian Brown's sleepless nights are not at all unusual.

One group, researching the moral concerns of families caring for children who had been receiving long-term ventilator assistance at home, was able to recruit only eleven families, in part because the families contacted had difficulty scheduling time for the home interview required. Of the eleven families, only three had time to schedule an additional, in-depth interview, so the study was based only on initial short interviews. The participating families reported, "Virtually every aspect of their lives was highly complicated and frequently overwhelming" (Carnevale et al., 2006, p. e53).

Ventilator-dependent children are possibly among the sickest and most labor-intensive of children who can be sent home from the hospital. Many of them require full-time observation because even a temporary malfunction of the breathing apparatus can have disastrous consequences. However, the same research group also noted that families with less-ill children—those who did not require full-time ventilation or were able to receive support via face-mask rather than tracheostomy—were not significantly different or less distressed than those families whose children required full time ventilatory support via tracheostomy (Carnivale et al., 2006, p. e53). This is a very small sample and may not be relevant for other types of home health care, but it lends support to the idea that all families caring for medically complex children at home encounter similar significant problems.

Care is time-consuming and exhausting even for those children whose disabilities do not require support from home medical technology, however. Many children with special needs, particularly those with autism or other forms of intellectual disability, experience delays in development which prolong stages of infancy or childhood. The normal work of infancy—particularly feeding, dealing with nighttime crying, and changing diapers—can extend years or decades past the time it is usually necessary. The toddler years, during which children are active but are not yet aware of possible dangers in the environment, can also be extended indefinitely. This "parenting plus" (Ray, 2002) is a major factor in extreme caregiving.

Savannah, whom we met in this book's Preface, was diagnosed with CFC, the same syndrome as Walker Brown, in her teens. At nineteen years old, Savannah could feed herself, in the messy way of toddlers everywhere, smearing herself with pureed food and scattering crackers on the floor. Savvy had outgrown her need for continuous nighttime feedings via her gastrostomy tube, but she still needed her tube for her numerous medications and for fluid supplementation. She could walk and communicate a bit by sign language, but she was not toilet trained and frequently woke at night.

Every night at about eight, her father changed her diaper and rocked her to sleep, a task which had become more difficult over the years as she grew and gained weight. He went to bed when Savannah fell asleep and got up again when she did, at 4 AM. He bounced her in his arms continuously to keep her happy and quiet, until it was time for him to go to work. Annette always stayed up until midnight, when she had to change Savannah's diaper (and often bedding) before a predictably full diaper made Savvy uncomfortable enough to wake everyone up. Annette was up again at 6 AM to take over from Savvy's father and get her ready for her day program at school. After nineteen years of this, they were both exhausted.

Samuel, who has multiple impairments due to a syndrome called Cornelia DeLange syndrome, at age nine, was developmentally ahead of Savannah. This did not necessarily make his parents' work any easier. Samuel could happily feed himself, though his milk needed to be thickened so he wouldn't choke on it, and he had to be prevented from stuffing too much food in his mouth at once. Needless to say, mealtime was rather messy. He usually went to bed without difficulty, but often woke at night and needed to be rocked back to sleep. He was not toilet trained, though it was beginning to look as though some day he might achieve this. Accidents were frequent and sometimes compounded by Samuel's desire to "help" clean up. An active nine-year-old who doesn't want his diaper changed can, if nothing else, vastly increase the number of infant-sized wipes consumed per diaper.

Samuel's most time-intensive problems, though, arose from his mobility. He loved opening and closing things: cabinets, toilets, doors, windows. As he grew, he learned to defeat ever more complicated latches. He was fearless—and clueless. He had no idea that he might be hurt by falling out the window or running in front of a car. Essentially, an adult had to watch him every moment that he was awake, ready to keep him away from the street, pull him off the bookshelves, or prevent him from climbing over the back fence and running away. And he was fast. One day when I was visiting the family as a friend, I chased him as he ran into a neighbor's house and, since he wouldn't come when called, physically pulled him back outside. While I was closing their door, he disappeared. After five minute's search, he had not been found. We thought of all the places he could reach in five minutes—a nearby lake, the highway, a little woods. The police were on their way when we found him. He had made his way back through the neighbor's house into their garage, where he was playing in their car.

The neighbors found him when they went to investigate the reason their garage door was mysteriously going up and down.

Dangerous behavior is not the only problem caused by motility, however. We call the toddler years the "terrible twos" because it is a constant battle against chaos. Meals are messy. Clothes need to be changed frequently, and it takes much longer to dress a child who can remove clothing faster than a caregiver can put it on. A child with a short attention span will zoom between activities; pushing buttons on a toy, then turning a few pages of a book, then emptying the contents of a toy chest or a kitchen drawer. The verbal toddler is also known for incessant demands. I very much admire the parents who can answer a question like "Go Grampa's now?" with the same patient, cheery answer, as though it hadn't been asked a hundred times that day. "No, we are driving up to Grandpa's farm for a visit in two weeks." Even conversation can be wearing, particularly if the toddler can physically get in the way until answered.

However, an example of perhaps the most intense work of caring for a child with special needs is found in Ann Fadiman's book *The Spirit Catches You and You Fall Down* (1997). This book is frequently included in medical school curricula, but it is most commonly used to demonstrate the need for cultural sensitivity. The book is about a child named Lia Lee, who had an intractable seizure disorder. Misunderstandings between Lia's American doctors and her Hmong immigrant parents led to a delay diagnosing an episode of overwhelming sepsis and meningitis when Lia was four years old. The book details the problems encountered in treating Lia's seizures and emphasizes the different ways in which the Hmong culture views health and medicine. Though this is not a parent caregiving memoir, Fadiman's keen observations include many clues to the sort of caregiving that Lia's mother performed.

Following her disastrous illness at age four, Lia was unable to move purposefully, swallow voluntarily, or respond to sight and sounds. The doctors expected her to die when she was sent home from the hospital, but she did not, mostly due to her mother's extraordinary caregiving. Lia Lee lived in a persistent vegetative state, at home under her mother's care, until her death in 2012 at age thirty (Fox, 2012).

Lia's mother, Foua, rejected all the technology later offered by her medical team. Lia was not tube fed, though any other child in the same state would have been. Her parents removed Lia's NG tube after a week, because it frequently became plugged by the food they were trying to force through it. The book describes how Foua managed to feed her, at first by "squeez[ing] formula into her mouth with a baby bottle" (Fadiman, 1997,

p. 212), then later by pre-chewing food for Lia, or grinding it up with a mortar and pestle, before putting it in her mouth. Fadiman says,

> Every day Foua boiled quantities of a spinach-like vegetable called *zaub*, which she grew specially for Lia in the parking lot, and fed her the broth. Lia usually straddled Foua's lap, her long legs sticking out on either side, while Foua, after putting her lips to the food to make sure it wasn't too hot, coaxed tiny bites into her mouth. She always wiped Lia's drool with her hand rather than with a napkin or a towel. "It takes a long time to eat," she told me [Fadiman] once, as she fed Lia rice. "You have to open Lia's mouth to look inside, because if there is already rice in there and you put some more in, she might vomit it back out. You have to hold your hand in back of her neck all the time or she can't swallow." Then she laughed and kissed Lia's ricey mouth. (1997, p. 217)

Foua would not use the expensive wheelchair provided, preferring to carry Lia everywhere in a "*nyias*," a Hmong baby carrier, which she made herself. "It was perhaps the largest *nyias* in Hmong history, since Lia was more than three feet tall and weighed thirty-six pounds," says Fadiman (p. 210). Lia slept with Foua instead of in the hospital bed acquired with some difficulty by a social worker. "'Lia always sleeps with us,' Foua told me. 'She is the only child who sleeps in our bed. I hold her during the night and we pat her feet all night long because we love her so much. If you don't pat Lia on her foot or her knee, she cries a lot'" (p. 212–213). Lia was fifteen when Fadiman's book was published. Her mother, whose birth date in a hut in the mountains of Laos is unrecorded, was in her late fifties at that time and over seventy when Lia died.

Extreme caregiving for Lia must have been an enormous task, and, unlike typical parenting, the need for care did not diminish with time. As with the parents in Lynne Ray's study, Foua had to continue to care for Lia as though she was an infant for an extended period. But such "parenting plus" is not merely a prolongation of infancy. Many of the tasks that need to be done for infants are more daunting and time-consuming in an older child. One mother of a sixteen-year-old with severe cerebral palsy and major intellectual delays reminded me that changing a diaper does not have the same meaning for her as for many mainstream parents. Her son's hip is dislocated, his knee contracted, and his shoulder subluxed due to his dystonia. She needs to vent his G-tube while changing his diaper, leaving it open so that if he vomits in agitation, his stomach contents will come out of the tube rather than his nose and mouth. The task of changing her son's diaper, though it goes by the same name, is much different, more complex, and more time-consuming than the simple task of changing an infant.

The very fact that children get bigger and taller as they grow up intensifies some of the challenges of caring for them. Children with behavior outbursts, common in severe autism, grow strong enough to deal disturbingly large amounts of physical damage: leaving holes in walls, breaking windows and, occasionally, causing bodily injury to themselves or caregivers. Children with bone diseases might lose mobility as increasing size leads to inability to support their own weight or as the curvature of their spine increases with growth. Some children actively resist care because it is uncomfortable; as when muscle spasticity diminishes thigh movement or the touch of a diaper wipe burns sensitive skin. If a somewhat mobile older child doesn't want to cooperate with a diaper change or bath, the child must be held in place while the task is done, leaving fewer hands free for working. These simple activities then require either a good deal of manual dexterity or the presence of more than one caregiver.

For many profoundly developmentally delayed or neurologically impaired children, increasing body weight alone poses an enormous challenge. Like Lia Lee, some children remain permanently confined to bed and wheelchair. Yet an adult-sized child must be moved to prevent bed sores or to perform daily hygiene. They must be carried from bed to bath and supported while in the tub. In order for them to leave their rooms, their parents must dress them and move them to the new location. Some of these increased needs can be met by already available, simple technology, such as wheelchairs and lifts (Rizzo, 2014). But, of course, transferring a child from bed to lift, and lift to wheelchair, transforms an act of carrying that is both intimate and brief into a complicated, mechanized effort.

In addition, parent-caregivers become less physically capable as they age, less able to carry a heavy child from room to room, or lift two long legs in order to wipe between them. Both Savannah and Samuel have short statures and low weight as part of their syndromes, but the day will come when Savannah's father can no longer rock her to sleep in his arms and Samuel's mother will not be able to run faster than he does. It comes as no surprise that researchers find that as both parents and children age, concern about how their children's special needs will be met in the future multiplies (Ray, 2002; Carnevale et al., 2006). Extreme caregiving is physically exhausting and, unless the child makes major developmental progress, often becomes more difficult as time goes on.

Financial Burden

Noah Greenfeld was born in 1966, the second son of Josh Greenfeld and Foumi Kometani. Josh was a self-employed writer, the author of several novels and screenplays, and Foumi was a writer and painter. At first everything was fine, and the journal Noah's father kept was filled with mundane concerns about the increasing expense of having two children and needing to move to a larger house. But when Noah reached nine months, his doctor noticed that Noah was not meeting the expected developmental milestones. This began a long, difficult, and often expensive journey to discover what, if anything, was wrong with Noah, and what, medically, could be done about it.

Greenfeld published his diary of Noah's first five years, *A Child Called Noah* (1970), shortly after Noah's final diagnosis of autism. At the time, autism was even less well understood than it is now, and Noah had been through a number of diagnoses, including "classic retardation," "brain damage," and childhood schizophrenia. He'd been seen by pediatricians, neurologists, psychologists, speech therapists, and chiropractors at several hospitals and research institutes. Meanwhile, at home, Noah had temper tantrums, outbursts of unexplained laughter and crying, and stopped talking or trying to communicate in any way other than screaming.

The therapies his parents tried were many, varied, and time-intensive. They tried a brief stint of "patterning," which was popular in the sixties, and requires several adults to force a child to crawl for hours a day. They tried mega-vitamin therapy, special diets, a variety of classes developed for children or adults with behavior problems, and programs to treat what was then called retardation. At one point, despite some financial hardship, the entire family moved to California to participate in a new program of behavior modification called "operant conditioning." All this expense and effort earned Noah the ability to use the toilet most of the time, help dress himself, and feed himself. He did not learn to name colors, count to ten, or talk.

Foumi was in charge of maintaining the daily routine of caregiving, spending her time at home or at one of a succession of expensive private schools, implementing whatever behavior program they were currently trying. Because of the time she spent finding and taking Noah to these programs, as well as controlling Noah's behavior at home, she had to put her own career as writer and painter on hold. Josh meanwhile found an office away from home and the disruptions caused by Noah's outbursts, though his career as a screenwriter still suffered. Josh laments the loss of time dedicated to his own writing and the cessation of Foumi's creative activities, as well as the limitation of time and attention given to Noah's older brother Karl.

Ironically, it was Noah who indirectly provided both the literary inspiration his parents needed and the financial capital for some of his later care. *A Child Called Noah* was an immense success. It was one of the earliest books about raising a child with autism, and for a brief time the Greenfelds were minor celebrities. There were numerous articles and interviews, and an appearance on *60 Minutes* (Greenfeld, 2009; Morrice, 2009). It was followed by two other books, *A Place for Noah* in 1978 (diaries from 1971–1977) and *A Client Called Noah* in 1986 (1977–1980) covering Noah's life from age five to fourteen. His mother, Foumi, wrote a fictionalized story about a child much like Noah, which was published in Japan to much literary acclaim. Even Noah's brother, Karl Taro Greenfeld later wrote a book about Noah. *Boy Alone* was published in 1990 and added some new details to Noah's teenage years as well as following him into adulthood.

Toward the end of *A Child Called Noah*, Greenfeld (1970), observes cynically, "Indeed, the more I read about such children, the more I'm convinced, unfortunately, that only money can solve most of the problems of having a child like Noah. That's the damned truth of it. The more money I have, the less of a problem Noah becomes—I can hire out the problem to others. Have a crazy kid and get to understand the gut meaning of society" (pp. 126–127). The family spent much of the money they made from the success of *A Child Called Noah* on educational programs and care for Noah.

It is not surprising to find that families raising children with special needs, particularly those with multiple medical problems, often encounter financial difficulties. A US national survey of children with "medical complexity," defined as receiving chronic treatment from multiple specialists, showed that 50% of families reported that health care for their child had caused financial problems (Thomson et al., 2016). Another study, on a subset of children with special health care needs (CSHCN) whose needs were considered more significant, found that 57% of families reported financial difficulty (Kuo et al., 2011). While some of the expense may be due to lack of proper medical insurance, several studies of families of technology-dependent children in Canada, England, and Australia—countries that provide universal health care—also revealed significant financial difficulties because so much of what the families needed was not covered by universal health care (Wang & Bernard, 2004; Kirk, 1998; Cockett, 2012).

In the United States, where we are now just beginning to attempt universal coverage, both direct and indirect costs can be expected. A representative survey done in Minnesota in 1998, on families receiving TEFRA, Minnesota's supplementary health coverage for medically complex children, found that the average annual medical cost for a child on TEFRA (in 1998) was $35,000, of which only 77% was covered by various insurances. Families on TEFRA were spending about 11% of their income on medical care for their child with disabilities, while the average spent by families without a disabled child was 5.5% (Chan et al., 1998). The out-of-pocket expense of medical bills, home equipment, therapy, and home health care nurses will, of course, vary wildly depending on insurance coverage and diagnosis. But we can assume that this increased expenditure takes its financial toll on most, if not all, families doing extreme caregiving in the United States.

Even with the best of coverage, there are hidden expenses. One study of technology-dependent children reported, "equipment, pharmaceutical, electricity, telephone and transport expenses are potential financial burdens that are hidden within families" (Wang & Bernard, 2004, p. 41). Doctor and hospital visits might be covered by insurance, but travel expenses and the time taken off from work to get to them usually are not. Perhaps the large-sized diapers and the special formulas are covered, but not always. Durable medical equipment, such as ventilators or the pumps for continuous tube feeding, is often covered, but gloves, tape, and other supplies needed to maintain them may not be. Nor are some ordinary things—like safety locks needed well past the typical toddler years, gates that will keep a toddler in a nine-year-old-size body safe, or toys that might interest an unreachable child with autism. An unusual piece of equipment, such as a GPS to locate a child who frequently runs away, might be covered by a special grant, but there is a waiting period, and the amount of paperwork required to document its necessity can be mountainous.

Insurance companies do not always view with kindness the expenses that can be incurred by a child with complex medical problems. Deanna Fei recounts her experiences following the birth of her daughter at 25-1/2 weeks (5-1/2 months) in her memoir *Girl in Glass* (2015). Just as Fei and her daughter were recovering from the harrowing NICU stay, the company where Fei's husband worked announced significant cuts in employee benefits. The CEO of the company claimed that the reason for the cuts was that they had paid a million dollars to save Fei's "distressed baby." Fei found herself at the center of a media firestorm, suddenly called upon to defend her child and others who had been accused of using more than their fair share of medical resources. Her husband left the company at the first opportunity, with no financial loss. But many others contacted Fei reporting that they had lost jobs and/or medical insurance following serious illnesses or high-risk pregnancies (Fei, 2015).

An additional, unmeasured financial burden comes from the frequent need for parents to take time off from work or reduce work hours. Sixty-four percent of the parents on TEFRA responded that their employment was affected in some way, with the most frequent response being "accepted a lower paying job with more flexibility or fewer demands" (Chan et al., 1998, p. 3). It is not unusual, if the child's needs are intense, for one or both parents to have to quit their jobs. In the national survey of families of children with special health care needs (CSHCN), researchers found that 22% of parents reduced their work hours, and 20% stopped working, about twice the rate reported by families whose children did not have special health care needs (Romley, 2017). This data was based on a broad definition that included many families that were not doing extreme caregiving, however. Researchers who evaluated a subset of families of CSHCN, whose children had increased need due to complex medical problems, found that 54% reported a family member who had to stop working because of the child's health problems (Kuo, 2011). Researchers working with the families of technology-dependent children likewise mention the frequent need for one parent to have to quit working, and found that this parent is usually the mother (Kirk, 1998; McKeever & Miller, 2004; Cockett, 2012).

As a pediatrician, I did not encounter many situations where lack of insurance coverage for illnesses was a major problem. Though I do not know that this is true in every state, various federal and state programs, such as TEFRA, seemed willing to step in and provide additional coverage for children with chronic medical problems. Instead, I saw families, even those with excellent insurance coverage, struggling to meet the uncovered expenses. Most of the families of children with special needs that I have followed found themselves in difficult financial straits at some point. Two were forced to declare bankruptcy, in part due to the combination of medical and home health care expenses with loss of income from one parent. None of the families with two working parents were able to continue sustaining a dual income after their child's needs became apparent; most often it was the mother who had to quit her job.

Health care providers and insurance companies often assume that caring for medically complex, chronically ill, or technology-dependent children at home is the most cost-effective way to provide care. Progress in home-care technology is in part motivated by evidence that suggests that home care reduces costs. However, some scholars have pointed out that the financial, social, and emotional costs to families usually are not taken into account in calculations of expenses. It is likely that most of the reduction in medical expenses that results from home care is due to "the substitution of parental for professional nursing care," which comes at a high cost in terms of stress to parents (Kirk, 1998, p. 104). A recent cost analysis of caregiving for all children with special health care needs (CSHCN) estimated that it would cost about $12 billion dollars to replace family caregivers with unskilled laborers, and $36 billion to provide skilled labor (Romley, 2017). It is likely that if the cost of parental caregiving were taken into account, home care would not be less expensive than institutional care.

Acknowledging that there are financial costs attendant to home care for children with disabilities, some researchers have suggested ways to mitigate families' financial hardship. One researcher recommended that home care programs "should require significant family supports in the way of salary support, provision of part-time assistance within the home, and the development of suitable respite services" to reduce financial strain on the family (Carnevale et al., 2006, p. e59). Others pointed out that readily available health care coordinators and internet databases of available services would also serve as steps toward easing the burdens on the family. However, without measurements of the actual hands-on caregiving work required, the beneficial effects of any of these efforts are not quantifiable (Ray, 2002, pp. 435–436). I believe that assigning random families the burden of extreme caregiving while refusing to acknowledge and support the additional financial burden is an obvious wrong that needs to be addressed as soon as possible.

Families also have experienced difficulty in acknowledging that they need financial help. One mother, writing largely in order to cope with her own feelings, observed that many parents of children with special needs like herself struggled to accept help because they were used to thinking of themselves as "self-sufficient people" who could "maintain control" over their lives. She found it "devastating" to realize that she had to accept financial assistance from governmental programs for the disabled to meet her daughter's medical needs (Jennings, 1995). Asking for assistance can feel like it undermines a parent's status as an independent, contributing member of society. For this mother, the shame that stemmed from this impression compounded the emotional tolls of daily life, adding to the exhaustion of providing for the needs of her child at home.

When a parent-caregiver is forced to give up employment, that parent loses a source of status and fulfillment, as well as income. While caregiving involves a tremendous amount of work, society does not afford the same respect to family care work as it does to conventional full-time employment. Despite feminist gains that allowed women to join the workforce, caregiving, particularly family caregiving, has yet to be recognized as a valid and worthy career. When feminism claimed that women's work no longer had to be in the home, it had the unfortunate side effect of suggesting that work outside the home is more worthy, contributing to the feeling that care work is of less consequence (Tronto, 1993). Parents rarely mention this particular challenge, perhaps due to their tendency to think in terms of the needs of their child and not their own, but some parents, both mothers and fathers, do experience the loss of their jobs as diminishing a crucial part of their identity. The loss of a career, or even a paying job, thus becomes a personal and a financial crisis.

Linda had to quit her job to take care of her son Samuel. She regretted not only losing her income, though that was a considerable blow, but also losing a job that she loved. She was good at it, she said, able to organize others and get projects done on time. She was very proud that during the years she worked, she increased efficiency enough that she was able to do the work of several employees. But she had to quit because raising Samuel required all of her time. She was very good at that too. All the skills she had demonstrated in her job were just as apparent at home. Her caregiving for Samuel was a marvel of kindness, patience, and holding onto a modicum of organization against the whirlwind of Samuel's constant motion. Yet, though her pride in Samuel's accomplishments was evident, she did not often speak with pride of her own contribution to his success.

It seemed odd to me that Linda would think more highly of her organizational skills at work than at home nurturing a child. Perhaps you could explain this from an economic viewpoint; her family was indeed struggling financially without her paycheck. Linda reported that positive feedback at work was the determining factor in her confidence. At work there were defined goals, and rewards when they were accomplished. She could tell when she had done a good job. But with Samuel, there were no rules, and no way to measure success. It doesn't really matter what Linda's old job was, but I find it particularly ironic. She worked at a printing company that fulfilled orders for mass-mail advertisements. Yet she felt more comfortable about her competence producing junk mail than she did when she turned to caring for her child full time. We will return to this topic in the chapter on competence.

The need to provide caregiving for their children with disabilities obviously curtails and shapes the careers of many parents, particularly the mothers, no matter their chosen professions. Very few parents are able to supplement either the income or the self-esteem lost from having to give up a regular job. Adding to this strain, the parents must assume uncovered medical expenses, even if they have the best medical insurance. Like the Greenfelds, who experienced financial difficulties despite the income provided by their brief celebrity, many extreme caregiving parents find it difficult to keep up.

Social Isolation

Charles Hart's son Ted was born in 1974 and, like Noah Greenfeld, developed problems that were not immediately identifiable. Ted could read and talk and memorize things, but his ability to use the facts he could recite remained elusive. He was not toilet trained successfully, and he did not sleep at night. After years of receiving misdirected diagnoses from professionals, Hart himself diagnosed Ted with autism after hearing about autism at a teacher's conference. Ted's doctors then admitted that they had been deliberately shielding the family from this presumed-terrible diagnosis, but for Hart the knowledge was a relief. At that point, Ted was ten years old, and Hart had resigned from his job as a hospital administrator in training. In addition to caring for his son, he became an advocate for autism programs and research, working with state grant money. Hart chronicled his life with his son in the memoir *Without Reason: A Family Copes with Two Generations of Autism* (1989).

The first "generation of autism," referred to in the book's title, was Hart's much older brother Sumner. Sumner had been born in 1929 at a time when most parents of children with developmental delays chose to institutionalize them, but their mother had refused to do this. She lived her whole life for Sumner, rarely going outside, in order to shelter him from condescending eyes, and to shelter herself from the shame of bearing him. She had accepted Sumner's differences as an untransferable burden, with the hope of outliving him her only plan for the future. Hart writes, "Widowed and living alone with an eccentric son, she was socially isolated. Their small apartment became a prison as arthritis and osteoporosis further restricted her activity" (1989, pp. 123–124). She continued to watch over Sumner, both of them trapped in her home, until her death. By that time, Sumner was over fifty and had been living in isolation with his mother since birth. We will return later to the problems this caused for him.

Hart also had to unlearn some of the lessons regarding the supposed shame of disability that he learned from his mother's example. As a young man, and again as a young father, Hart reported spending a lot of time apologizing for, or attempting to control, embarrassing or inappropriate behaviors from his brother and, later, his son. He understood this as a way to protect them. But neither Sumner nor Ted were equipped to notice public shame. As part of their autism, they never saw or responded to the emotions of others. Eventually, Hart realized that he was doing this, not to protect them from humiliation, but to protect himself. "Protect Ted? Protect Sumner?" he asks. "Slowly I had to recognize that a sense of family shame made me want to hide them, protecting *me* from public judgment as surely as I tried to conceal them from their imaginary persecutors" (1989, p. 264). That there is no need for such shame does not make the feeling any less real for him or the isolating consequences any less difficult.

In recent years, the shame imposed by society on Sumner Hart's mother, and on my parents as well, for bearing a child with disabilities, has lessened. Yet parents of children with special needs continue to feel isolated from their friends and relatives. Families of chronically ill children report that close friends and even family members often drift away after initially offering support (Ray, 2002; Kirk, 1998). Almost all the papers on caring for technology-dependent children indicate that parents report feeling social isolation, and the papers cite a number of different reasons why this is so. Many families describe essentially becoming house-bound because they are simply too exhausted to go elsewhere. They have difficulty finding respite care and fear leaving their child with complex problems to someone else's care. Some are reluctant to have guests because of the intimidating nature of the changed home environment, taken over by medical equipment and home health care nurses (Kirk, 1998). The home can be transformed into a medical space that operates around the clock. Not everyone who comes to visit knows how to react when they see medical equipment in the child's bedroom or tube feedings as part of a family meal. The home can also become a public space, visited frequently by strangers. Few understand the etiquette for interacting with home health care workers who are not family or friends, and yet whose work is an intimate part of the household proceedings.

Some researchers claim that social isolation results from a failure of social services to provide adequate support (Wang & Bernard, 2004). Everyone who has worked with children with special needs, I suspect, would agree that the current level of support provided to children and their parents is inadequate. Access to those services that are available is sometimes complicated by an overwhelming and time-consuming amount of paperwork (Ray, 2002). In addition, when families are offered "support," it often comes in the form of counseling or therapy, which for many families just adds another appointment to their already full schedule.

In 1999, the Finnish nursing scholar Berit Brinchmann conducted long interviews in the homes of seven families who were (or had been) living with a severely disabled child (two of the children had since died). Most of the parents described exhaustion, sleeplessness, and sorrow, leading to feelings of loneliness and being trapped in the home. Brinchmann wrote, "The home can seem like a prison, from which it is impossible to escape" (1999, p. 137), echoing Charles Hart's description of his mother's decades-earlier caregiving for his autistic brother Sumner.

Much of the social isolation these parents experience is not imposed by the amount and difficulty of work involved, but by the way disability is viewed in society. Sumner's mother in the 1930s and 1940s was trapped by a perceived societal standard that said that a parent who bore a disabled child must feel a sense of shame, and that those who made the somewhat foolhardy choice to keep their child at home must hide the child from others. The expectation that parents protect the world from differences by hiding their children has perhaps abated, along with the shame imposed. But parents still hear stories of disparaging comments made in public places, such as a comment, overheard in a WalMart by the parent of a child with Cornelia DeLange syndrome: "Those deformed children shouldn't be born." They hear reports of bullying of children who don't fit in for any reason and feel a need to stay home with their children to protect them from a disapproving world.

My mother reports that my brother's elementary school classes in the late 1960s were held in tiny, windowless rooms, with doorways covered in brown paper even though they were tucked as far away as possible from the active hallways. Principals and teachers casually informed my parents that the occupants of this classroom were not quite students, and that their presence might be somehow damaging to the "real" children. Great effort was expended to ensure that they were never visible to the other students in hallways or on the playground. I have no memories of the location or appearance of my brother Paul's classrooms, and Paul's twin remembers no interactions with him at school. We did not realize that this was an intentional policy at the time.

The church was only slightly more forgiving. When I was a teenager, my parents suddenly changed churches. I later found out that a pastor told my parents that they could no longer bring my brother to his church, as it was disturbing to the other attendees. Since my brother at that point did very little except sit and drool, and had never been disruptive, the minister could only have been objecting to his obvious disability. Happily, another church, only a bit further away, was amenable to starting a Sunday school class for children who had been diagnosed with "mental retardation." My brother attended classes there for years after, and their events and dances became the center of his social life and the introduction to lifelong friendships.

My parents' battle for appropriate education for my brother slowly wore away at the pervasiveness of this segregation. Today's parents (and their children, both with and without disabilities) benefit from the success of early advocacy for the rights of children with disabilities, but there is still a need for progress. In Chapter 5, I return to the question of parents as advocates for their children, and the persistence of forms of stigma and devaluation.

Even in these enlightened times, families report the need to protect their children and themselves from disapproving eyes. In a 2006 study, parents reported feeling isolated from their families who disapproved of their decision to keep their child at home. One family with two children with disabilities reported avoiding public places like the mall because the "stares" from strangers made them uncomfortable (Carnevale et al., 2006, p. e56). A mother of a child with Velocardiofacial syndrome, associated with behavior problems due to childhood psychosis, wrote, "Other people . . . have steadily helped me into isolation. Family, friends, spouse, the person in front of you at the grocery store—they'll tell you he behaves like he does because you are too strict, too lax, too distant, too pampering. They aren't trying to be cruel; they want to help" (Carver, 2007, p. 35). More recently, mothers of children with disabilities reported that they have been the targets of direct disapproval from strangers. They stated that they receive hostile stares and remarks, particularly if their child has a "meltdown" or behaves atypically in public. A nursing scholar and mother of a child with severe autism reported that, even in 2014, she "continued to be met with disapproval, criticism, and unwarranted advice from family members and strangers" (Zibricky, 2014, p. 45).

One of the ways to combat these less-than-helpful stares and comments is to maintain the appearances of normality when in public. If parents cannot succeed in making their children "pass" as typical because of an unmistakable disability or unusual behavior, they sometimes try to compensate by being very conscious of their children's hygiene and dress. Sociologists McKeever and Miller (2004) noted that mothers of disabled children reported investing a lot of time and effort into keeping their children not only meticulously clean but also fashionably and brightly dressed. The mothers in their study saw this attention to appearance not merely as a way to prove the adequacy of their care, but also primarily as a way to increase their child's social standing and, ultimately, value. Conforming to appearance in this way also helps parents endure the stares they inevitably receive, maintaining a personal wall against the disapproval or guilt they are sometimes made to feel.

This is not a new strategy. My brother lived at home into adulthood, and nearly every morning, before taking him to the sheltered workshop where he worked, my mother would send him back up to the bathroom to shave areas that he had missed on the first or, sometimes, second attempt. It was terribly frustrating for him, and mystifying to me. The spots he missed were essentially invisible next to his unsteady gait and slack mouth. My mother insisted that his cleanliness reflected the adequacy of the care she was providing. She was also, without realizing it, establishing his right to a presence in the world, by insisting on correctness in those things she could control.

Another reason that contact with the outside world is fraught for families with children with special needs is that every encounter with someone outside the family, whether it takes place inside or outside the home, can remind the parent of the disability, essentially breaking down the private world in which the child's problems become the norm. One researcher reports, "One family felt isolated by seeing their friends' children grow up, while their son with developmental delay did not: the universe moves on while the family feels stuck and left behind" (Carnevale et al., 2006. p. e56).

In many of the parent narratives, there is a moment when watching typical children causes sadness and perhaps a bit of unintended jealousy. Greenfeld (1970) describes a visit to friends with children the same ages as two-year-old, autistic Noah and his older brother Karl. He writes,

> It's getting painful to watch children grow past Noah. This afternoon we dined with some friends whose two-year-old son joined—or followed after—Karl . . . in play, while Noah just sat on the couch or in the corner, addressing his fingers and grinding his teeth. The same thing happened

> Thanksgiving Day. Other friends were over with their three kids. Their baby girl, a little thing, now talks, while Noah remains a baby. (p. 126)

Contact with strangers, or even friends, is not without consequence, even when there is no criticism. It can be a reminder of the widening gap in development between their child and the typical child, knowledge that often must be put aside to get through an ordinary day.

The essay "Welcome to Holland" mentions this briefly. Kingsley warns parents who arrive unexpectedly in Holland, rather than in Italy, not to compare their child with the child they thought they would have. If they spend too much time regretting the loss of a typical child, they will miss the wonderful things about the child they have. But it is hard not to be blindsided by Italy, when a child such as Noah Greenfeld spends time with an age mate and is so obviously delayed. It may be easier to stay home than to risk a sudden reminder of the things the disabled child is likely to miss.

Interestingly, in one of the most recent parenting autobiographies, *The Boy in the Moon*, Ian Brown (2011) claims to have no problems when he and his son are out in public. "The opinion of other people matters less and less the more you walk down the street with a boy whose lumpy looks attract attention, stares and smiles alike," he writes (p. 36). He does not discuss his wife's experiences, which may be quite different. Yet Brown recognizes that he is living a life that is very different from what his acquaintances are living, which leads him to reorder his priorities. He says, "The boy recalibrates the world. The crisis of so-and-so's unhappiness about her job or his inability to meet a woman who will pay him what he considers to be a sufficient degree of attention pales next to the crisis of how to stop Walker from beating his own brains out" (p. 36).

This reordering of priorities is indeed one of the benefits of living in Holland, yet Brown still feels isolated. Walker is too much work, too complicated, to leave with a babysitter. There is no nearby family, and the friends who do offer help rarely do so twice. And though he does not hide Walker from people, he is not entirely comfortable either. Walker is an active child, who interrupts conversations with his constant needs and who often physically intrudes on other's space. "He was a steady reminder not just of his presence, but of the existence of all children like him, the children we so often try to forget," Brown writes, then adds with his usual wry understatement, "For this reason we tended to select our dinner guests carefully" (p. 71).

I suspect that the need to carefully select one's friends, and even family, is the most isolating aspect of raising any child with special needs. For some, the changed atmosphere in the home is an obstacle to visitors. For others, their differently set priorities make social interaction less fulfilling. Although society has become more evolved in its attitudes toward people with disabilities since the time Sumner Hart was a child (or indeed since my brother was growing up), and the homes of families of children with severe disabilities need no longer feel like prisons, they can and do still feel shut off from the outside world. Home can be a safe haven, where there is a new and painstakingly constructed version of normality. Intrusions from the outside world can break it open. The careful selection of dinner guests and, more significantly, of viable family ties and friendships is, indeed, terribly important and potentially limits the social lives of extreme caregivers.

Silencing Negativity

One of my more distressing childhood memories of growing up with a "mentally retarded" brother comes from the early seventies. My brother would have been about eleven and attending classes at public school. Both of my parents were working hard to improve the education that he was receiving.[3] My father attended various meetings several times a month and seemed to enjoy them. He usually came home bragging about his part in the progress made. But one night he came home from a meeting of the Montgomery County Association for Retarded Children (MARC), an organization in which my parents were active members, enraged almost to the point of tears.

Most of the members of the MARC were fellow parents, and part of the meeting involved sharing their experiences. The other parents all expressed how wonderful it was, and how blessed they felt, to have the gift of a child with mental retardation. My father found this attitude unbelievable. He was at a loss for words at their misunderstanding but had finally managed

---

[3] My brother's right to an education had been legally established in 1966 when the Elementary and Secondary Education Act of 1965 was expanded to include "handicapped children," but the actual classes available to him were still inadequate. In the early 1970s the Montgomery County Association for Retarded Children (MARC) was supporting lawsuits against schools that excluded some children with intellectual disabilities through the Pennsylvania Association for Retarded Children (PARC). These cases dealt with exclusions of retarded children from public school, and are considered landmarks toward the passage of Public Law 94-142, the federal Education for All Handicapped Children Act of 1975 (Wright, 2010).

to blurt out, "It is not a gift. Mental retardation is Hell." His remark had angered the other members, which he found a shocking betrayal by people he thought he knew and trusted. He was still shaking with rage as he told us about it at home. He stated, repeatedly, "Mental retardation is Hell."

At the time, I completely understood my father's frustration. He was remembering the disappointments in Paul's first few years and the enormous effort it took for him to exceed the doctors' predictions that he would never walk or talk. He was resenting the times Paul's presence had limited our vacation options or turned a fifteen-minute walk into a two-hour ordeal. Perhaps these were merely selfish complaints, but underlying them was the nature of Paul's impairments. My father was a man who valued intelligence above all else, and he had been handed a son who had very little of it. He could not conceive of this as either a blessing or a gift.

I can now understand also the anger that his negativity must have provoked in the other parents at the meeting. My father had admitted to being unhappy about having a disabled son and complained that it made his own life Hell. The other parents had not only accepted their child's disabilities but also learned to recognize and value the good things those disabilities brought to their lives. Likely it had been a hard lesson, and none of them was completely comfortable in it. They had become special parents of special children, and any denial of that specialness seemed to threaten the value of both their lives and that of their children. For them, my father's remark was both untrue and completely unwelcome. It negated what they believed in and who they were trying to be. I imagine that other parents went home that night near tears, reminded unexpectedly of a grim reality in a place where they, too, had thought they were safe.

My father also did not realize that the fight to procure educational rights for "handicapped children" included a fight to acknowledge their existence as fellow human beings. As part of this, parents were desperately trying to make others understand the love they felt for their children and to establish their value to society. The congressional findings that emerged, following the actions of MARC and other parent groups, supported the education of children with disabilities in part because they hoped thus to create independent and productive citizens who could contribute to society (Wright, 2010). In revealing his frustration at my brother's lack of developmental progress, my father seemed to be publicly denying both the value of his son and the wisdom of trying to educate him. This not only called into question the other parents' coping strategies but also could be seen to undermine the legal process in which they were engaged.

The need to maintain a positive attitude, to sustain optimism in the face of adversity, might be a particularly American phenomenon. This emphasis on positive thinking seemingly produces a near requirement or duty to always look on the bright side (Ehrenreich, 2010; Sharot, 2011). It is so culturally ingrained that it colors, I believe, the entire experience of caring for a child with disabilities. This expectation is evident in online parent groups, where tips for parenting—discussions about which brands of diapers fit best, where to find special formula, and what gadget works best at capping a feeding tube—are mixed with cheeriness. To me, it sometimes feels as though parents are desperate to convince each other, and the world, how wonderful their children and their lives are.

The requirement for optimism is apparent also in the nature of the books published about special needs parenting, which seem to require, at the very least, a sunny acceptance and an insistence that, in the end, everything is for the best. According to narrative ethicist Howard Brody (2003) the preference for positivity is evident in books written about dealing with illnesses as well. Narratives by physicians and patients often end with the happy eradication of disease.

Brody states that there are three kinds of stories about illness: "redemptive," "chaos," and "quest" narratives. The first type is the most optimistic and the easiest to find. "Redemptive" narratives show the patient fighting their way through the challenges of illness and emerging triumphant and, usually, cured. Parent narratives of premature births, coming to grips with a diagnosis of Down syndrome, and finding personal cures for autism often follow this pattern. In my search for parent narratives, I found quite a few of these.

"Chaos" narratives, in which the life of the patient or parent cannot be organized into a coherent story arc, are rare because of their confusion and disorientation. The single chaos narrative that I found, a series of essays about trying to date while raising two sons with autism, managed to be optimistic through the use of a self-deprecating, black humor (Decker, 2011). Life, as one is living it, often seems like a chaos narrative. I have spoken to several parents who seemed comforted by the idea that life with children with autism is the definition of a chaos narrative, though perhaps not always funny. I think many other parents of kids with special needs might feel that their lives also fit this pattern.

It is the third type of narrative, the "quest" narrative, that Brody feels is the most useful sort of narrative for ethical analysis, and I agree. In the quest narrative, the patient or parent goes on a journey in response to illness or disability. They are seeking, not necessarily a cure, but a way to cope with a new way of life. Parents who report this journey do indeed report back from the unmapped territory of parenting children with special needs, to let us know what their lives are truly like. The parent brings testimony, not only to the child's challenges, but to the changes in his own life, and in himself, brought about by facing those challenges with the child.

Yet even in quest narratives, it is difficult to find parents willing to express the negative feelings my father reported. Many insist on maintaining positivity. Ian Brown (2011), interviewing parents of children with CFC, noted "a generally observed reluctance to complain or despair" (p. 135) and reports that he had to "coax" parents to describe the difficulties they encountered (p. 152).

In *Without Reason*, Charles Hart (1989) explains the benefit of a positive attitude to parents fighting to create a place in the world for their disabled child. He founded and attended an early autism parent support group, and states, "We tried to make the workshops a positive experience. Those parents needed more hope in their lives. They needed to feel positive about their handicapped children and to feel good about themselves as they struggled against social attitudes that tend to devalue people with disabilities and their parents" (p. 182). No doubt many in Hart's group benefited from the affirmation in overcoming the disapproval directed toward children with autism at the time. I wonder if anyone who complained too loudly was turned away. My father's experiences in the same decade demonstrate that not everyone was able to feel that positivity.

Helen Harrison (2001), a nurse and the mother of a child with disabilities, in a letter to the *Journal of the American Medical Association*, calls this expectation of positivity "Making Lemonade." She states that most parents feel the need to appear strong for other parents, their doctors, and even themselves. Those who do not can be seen as complainers, bad parents, or politically incorrect in their attitudes toward disability. She reports that parents who express negative feelings about their experiences or their child's disabilities have been forced out of support groups and banned from internet lists. She says, "Upon becoming parents of a disabled or 'high-risk' child, one of the first things we learn to do is lie—to our friends and family, to the doctors, to our child, and to ourselves. We quickly learn that others do not want an honest answer . . . and we oblige by giving the positive and politically correct answer" (Harrison, 2001, p. 239).

Harrison believes that this attitude is so pervasive that it calls into question the results of medical studies, particularly the quality of life studies done in Toronto under the direction of neonatologist Saroj Saigal. Her group has been following a cohort of NICU graduates who survived extremely premature births, questioning them about their physical health and their quality of life into the teenage years. For those children who had severe intellectual disabilities (about 6% of the participants), their parents answered the questions as proxies. In several later studies, teenagers with severe impairments and intellectual disabilities rated their quality of life higher than control teenagers on several scales, some of which, such as educational success, were clearly exaggerated (Saigal et al., 1996, 1999). Other studies have found that teenage survivors of premature birth, many of whom had significant health problems, rate their health-related quality of life as equal to or even better than their peers who have no diagnosed medical problems (Gray et al., 2007).

Based on the inconsistencies between actual and reported abilities, Harrison questions the reliability of these influential quality of life studies. She proposes that the parents and children involved in these studies felt that they had to give a positive report, knowing that it was their own doctors and hospital that were conducting the study. She feels that this inaccurately high assessment of the quality of life is a coping mechanism for dealing with severe disability, and reflects, among other things, a social mandate to be seen bearing up well under adversity, the need to maintain a politically correct attitude toward disability, and an unwillingness to disappoint the medical caregivers still actively involved with the child's care (Harrison, 2001).

I have observed that parents must walk a very tight line when interacting with medical or other professionals. They must unfailingly be seen to be coping well with the challenges. They must be champions for their child's needs and cheerleaders for their child's progress. This can mean hiding their own personal problems and minimizing the difficulties of caregiving. However, parents who hold an overly optimistic attitude, particularly about their child's prognosis in the face of a severe or life-limiting disability, can be labeled by their child's medical team as being "in denial," or unwilling to accept the reality of their child's disability. Sara Green, a disability scholar and mother of a daughter with cerebral palsy, confirms this. She reports that several studies have suggested "that parents who hold positive attitudes toward raising a child with a disability are often pathologized as being unrealistic, failing to accept their 'tragic' circumstances or being 'in denial' of their children's problems" (Green, 2006, p. 151). Rather than forgiving either parents or professionals for lapses in positivity, however, Green feels that parents must work to overcome negativity, and that this work increases the burden of caregiving. The line between excessive positivity and debilitating negativity seems to be drawn in different places by medical professionals and even other parents, which would make walking that line very hard indeed.

A perceived inequality between observed and reported quality of life has been reported in adult studies, where it has been called the "disability paradox." Not all agree that this is an actual paradox, but there have been numerous studies where adults with a variety of disabling conditions rate their quality of life unexpectedly high. In some of these studies, researchers find a tendency toward positivity but also suggest that maintaining positivity is a moral mandate.

Albrecht and Devlieger, early researchers of the so-called disability paradox, speculated that quality of life correlated with the ability of the disabled person to maintain a balance between body, mind, and spirit. They found that over half the people who self-identified as disabled reported a good quality of life. Those who reported a good quality of life felt that they were in control of their lives and coping well, had matured in their values and life goals, and had reached new definitions of success. Those who reported poor quality of life complained of distracting levels of pain, inability to cope, loss of control, and levels of fatigue that interfered with daily activities (Albrecht and Devlieger, 1999). Albrecht and Devlieger do not try to separate the characteristics that might result from a disabling condition from the characteristics of the disabled person themselves, however. Their results can be interpreted as evidence that a good quality of life and optimism seem to be related.

There are moral overtones, possibly unintentional, in Albrecht and Devlieger's findings. The terms applied to the possession of a good quality of life are all positive: coping well; strength in adversity; achieving a proper balance between body, mind, and spirit. A good quality of life implies a good person. To be fair, they do not actively suggest that a poor quality of life implies a bad person, but it is hard not to make this connection. Overcoming the stigma attached to disability and the winning of acceptance for people with disabilities become tied to maintaining a proper politically correct attitude toward disability. This is moral work. Those of us who are not disabled must realize that being disabled is perhaps not so bad. Those of us who are must then show the way by coping well, proving the theory by the example of their lives. It seems to me to add another burden to an already unfairly burdened life.

If, indeed, a paradox does exist in quality of life reporting, it might be explained by false reporting from people with disabilities, as Harrison believed. It could also indicate a lack of understanding of disability on the part of the group identified as nondisabled. Another series of investigations done on adults with disabilities found no evidence that people with disabilities were misreporting their experiences or exaggerating their satisfaction, however. Instead it seems that healthy, nondisabled people tend to be overly pessimistic about the effects of disabling conditions on people's lives. They also vastly underestimate the possibility of adaptation to new levels of ability (Ubel et al., 2005).

Both of these offer explanations of Saigal's findings that children with disabling conditions (sometimes aided by their parents) report a higher quality of life for themselves than expected. I suspect we are mis-imagining what a child's life with disabilities is truly like and underestimating the ability of children to adapt to circumstances. Saigal's studies were conducted by asking teens to rate the desirability of life with certain hypothetical disabling conditions. It may not be surprising that teens actively living with some of those same conditions rated life with them as more tolerable than did teens with no disability. Perhaps the only thing proven by the study of quality of life is that most teenagers and adults who are alive are happy to be so, no matter what their circumstances.

Fifty years later, my father's statement "Mental retardation is Hell" seems, at best, ill-considered and unkind. I do not think he ever understood that by saying he hated mental retardation, he seemed, to the other parents, to be negating the value of people who suffered from it. His scientific brain easily separated the diagnosis from the person affected by it, but the other parents must have heard him denying what they stood for. Yet I believe the feelings behind my father's statement were valid, and that he was not alone in feeling them. Because the other parents rejected him so quickly, that shared anger was never acknowledged or assuaged.

The lines my father crossed are even stronger now, and the silencing of transgressive voices is much more aggressive. There is, seemingly, a cardinal rule that makes public optimism toward disability a requirement for the parent of a child with disabilities. Expressions of anger toward the disability are considered tantamount to admitting an inability to accept and value the child. Those parents who cannot live by this maxim can be censured for their feelings, and support is withdrawn from the people who likely most need it. They must feel the same shame and loneliness that my father did. And so, like my father, they learn to hide their reservations, bury their anger, and never admit to needing help.

Ian Brown (2011) is one of the few writers who takes exception to the positive attitude expected from parent groups. Though he understands the importance of such reassurance, he and his wife abandoned support groups. In words that seem to echo my father's, he writes, "Walker had given my life shape, possibly even meaning. But Walker had also made our lives hell. On the hellish days the mawkish sermonizing about angels and specialness felt like rank self-delusion . . . .. It was hard to think of Walker as a gift from God, unless God was a sadist who bore a little boy a grudge" (pp. 135–136). I suspect he and my father would have understood each other well.

This culture of censure effectively silences the people who, like my father, admit to complaints or unhappiness. Their voices are hard to hear against a backdrop of optimism, and so, in this chapter, as well as in the rest of the book, I have tried to find quest narratives that relate all the realities of extreme caregiving. I admit to looking specifically for narrators who are willing to express the ambiguities of living with a child with multiple disabilities. I want to understand the anger my father had, the sadness underlying the care given to Lia Lee by her mother, and the odd loneliness expressed by Ian Brown.

Josh Greenfeld (1970), father of autistic Noah, writes, "I've leafed through three books, chronicles by parents of severely disturbed or brain damaged children. None of them palpitated with truth for me. The parents didn't burn with enough anger; they were all too damned heroic for me" (p. 126). Like him, I am searching for truths that are lost in the narrative of optimism and that many people are unwilling to voice.

I will return in Chapter 5 to the topic of overcoming stigma, which, we will see, clearly is a responsibility that parents of children with special needs must fulfill. They often become firm advocates for their child, insisting that a child will progress despite the doubts of others. They can become ardent, and sometimes strident, voices in the schools, in the political arena, and in promoting medical research into their child's disability. There, maintaining a positive attitude is also a nearly mandatory part of caregiving and carries its own burdens. But perhaps we cannot say that we truly have overcome stigma until everyone has an equal right to complain.

CHAPTER 4 | Narrative and the Phases of Care

WE HAVE SEEN that parents who care for children with a variety of disabilities at home have been given a physically challenging, financially burdensome, and emotionally value-laden task. These problems, identified by researchers in several fields, concur with some of the concerns expressed by parents in published narratives. While they are few in number, these parents potentially speak for tens of thousands of parents who are currently engaged in the task of extreme caregiving.

Some would say that by listening to the stories of these parents, we have already begun an ethical evaluation. Stories are a vital way of organizing and evaluating the world, and listening to unheard voices can reveal both unexpected truths and unsuspected problems. Narrative ethicist Howard Brody states, "Thinking about stories in this way is already to take an ethical stand, because to listen to a story, to enter into dialogue with the storyteller, is to decide to open oneself to the other's way of seeing the world" (Brody & Clark, 2014, p. s8). But, though we already might have begun to feel that extreme caregiving seems, at the very least, to be somewhat unfairly and randomly distributed, this is only the surface of the ethical work that needs to be done.

There are a number of systems for ethical analysis that have evolved over the past several decades. None of them have come up with universally definitive answers to some of medicine's most vexing questions, nor, I'm afraid, will I. I do believe, however, that the significant difference between various methods of doing ethics is not in the accuracy of their answers but in the sorts of questions they raise. We cannot find satisfying answers until we have uncovered new perspectives from which to look at problems and new ways of framing the questions that arise. One of the ways to do that is to examine narratives: individual, first-person accounts of people who have dealt with the dilemmas being considered.

Use of narrative in modern bioethics has its beginning in stories told by physicians about the practice of medicine; stories of the patients they encountered and the lessons they learned from those encounters. More recently, attention has turned to stories written by patients who bear direct witness to the suffering and humanity of bodily illness. Stories of sickness told by both professionals and patients have been important sources of understanding the body and mind in illness (Brody, 2003) and have contributed to our understanding of the ethics of such things as the doctor-patient relationship and dying with dignity (Frank, 2002).

In narratives written by people with disabilities or who have encountered illness, medical providers can discover the parts of the patient's life that the medical record leaves out. Stories of sickness can impart new understanding gained by living with pain or illness and offer guidance for people who are ill or may someday become ill. The ill storyteller offers the listener a testimony, a sort of living proof of another way of being, one that can benefit all of us, not just clinicians and patients. The narrative creates a moral community of listeners who share the experience. In this way, sick people who are willing to share their story are like travelers to a foreign country that we might expect to visit someday (Frank, 1995). The report they bring back can be a guidebook for that unexplored territory.

There are recognized problems with using stories as a basis for ethical decision-making, however. Even the proponents of narrative ethics realize that stories contain untruths, or at least distortions of the truth. These can be deliberate, as the author purposely slants the story to make himself look better or changes facts to produce a more engaging story. Or they can be subconscious if the author has unrecognized biases or prejudices. There is also no consistent basis upon which even the most truthfully told narrative can be identified as morally exemplary (Lindemann, 1997, 2004). However, despite some reservations based on the possibility of inaccuracy, unreliability, or social bias in the narrator, many now believe that narrative is, at the very least, a valid way to bring multiple voices into an ethical dialog (Arras, 1997).

Stories written by the parents of children with special health care needs or disabilities can likewise add dimension to our understanding of illness and disability. They fill important gaps by acknowledging the day-to-day challenges while also conveying the deep relationship between parent and child. They also can explore the moral and ethical questions that arise for the parent—not just those deemed important by the health care provider or ethicist.

Parents' stories differ somewhat from the usual medical stories of sickness, because the parents are neither versed in medicine nor physically affected themselves. This brings a new level of uncertainty to any information provided by such a narrative, since the parent is both interpreting the experience of another person and subject to the same unreliability as all narrators. But, though the disability resides in the body of the child, the parents are witnesses to it and to the unexpected ways of being it might bring about. By telling the story of caring for their child, the parent explains both what the child is going through and their own moral journey through unknown terrain. Their stories can provide rich nourishment for others who face similar challenges.

Narrative has been particularly useful for analysis of concerns that are situational or relational, or in which there are several potentially opposing points of view. It is perhaps the only way to undertake an analysis of the intimate, hidden relationship that is family caregiving. However, the narratives of parents are complex and multilayered, and if we are to uncover deeper ethical concerns, we need a framework within which to analyze them. In this chapter, I begin by outlining some of the sorts of questions that can be discovered using narrative. The majority of this chapter is spent on describing a system for analyzing caregiving from an ethical standpoint, which arises from the theories of political scientist Joan Tronto. To demonstrate the usefulness of her theories, I will introduce another parent narrative—the story that Vicky Forman tells about the lives and deaths of her premature twins in *This Lovely Life*.

A Narrative of Premature Birth

When Vicky Forman's twins were born at 23 weeks, over four months early, she begged the doctors to let them die. It was too soon, and she "knew these babies could not possibly survive or be normal if they did" (Forman, 2009, p. 6). She knew also that treatment in the NICU would be prolonged and intense, and she did not want them to suffer before they died. The doctors, however, told her that the babies would be born with signs of life, and that it was illegal not to resuscitate them. Within six hours, the twins were born and transferred to the NICU, where they received maximal treatment. The image of a peaceful ending in her arms, the deaths that Forman was denied, would haunt her ever after.

Forman persisted in her request for doctors to withdraw therapy but was not permitted even to instate a Do Not Resuscitate (DNR) order to refuse chest compressions in the event of cardiac arrest. However, within her first few days, one twin, Ellie, had a massive (grade IV) intra-cranial hemorrhage, which doctors felt would lead to death or severe, life-limiting disability. Forman persisted in her request to withdraw therapy and, on the fourth day in the NICU, based on Ellie's now-dismal prognosis, the doctors reluctantly granted her request. Ellie died in her arms a few hours later. Evan survived for almost eight years.

This is just the beginning of Forman's story, the beginning of her journey to become an extreme caregiver. Already she has had to face many of the difficult ethical challenges and decisions that have been raised by the success of neonatology at saving ever-smaller babies. I will return to her story after a brief review of the ethical complexities already revealed.

Under any system of ethics, Forman's decision for her premature infants poses a terrible and difficult dilemma. The twins were born in the so-called grey zone, the gestational ages between 23 and 25 weeks (average full-term is 40 weeks). At the time they were born, in 2000, survival in this zone was fairly low (around 50%) and the risk of moderate to severe disability was very high (around 80% of the survivors). For this reason, some neonatologists were reluctant to resuscitate these micro-preemies. Indeed Forman found out later that a nearby hospital had recently instituted a policy not to resuscitate before 25 weeks. Many neonatologists today still think that the risk is so great that the parents' wishes regarding resuscitation and treatment should be paramount or, at least, considered (Mercurio, 2005; Weiss et al., 2007; Wilkinson, 2011). But all are also aware of the so-called Baby Doe law, which states that doctors cannot withhold treatment from any child because of disabilities. This law is likely what Forman's doctors were thinking of when they told her that they could not legally withhold resuscitation for her twins.

Decisions such as these are often organized around the four principles of bioethics that were first proposed by philosophers Tom Beauchamp and James Childress in 1977. Their first principle, autonomy, recognizes and promotes a respect for persons as individuals, and includes a right to decide what happens to one's own body. In pediatrics, the right to make that decision is given to the parents, but, as I have said, that decision must be made entirely with the child's best interests in mind. In Beauchamp and Childress's system of ethics, parents must determine the child's interests by guarding their autonomy and balancing the remaining principles—beneficence, nonmaleficence, and justice.

Parents are usually considered to be the best judges of the child's best interests, and most do an excellent job at guarding them. However, not all parents will always consider their child's interests over their own, and so there is also a level of harm at which society must intervene. The ethical standard which was invoked when Vicky Forman presented in labor with twins at 23 weeks, was this "harm standard." If the babies were not resuscitated, they would die, and death is felt by many to be the ultimate harm. The mother's desire not to resuscitate could be overridden to prevent the harm of death.

In such a premature birth, with the likelihood of survival so low, treatment in the NICU might itself constitute a harm by prolonging the process of dying. Under the rubric of the principles of bioethics, the proper action is one in which benefit (beneficence) is maximized and harm (maleficence) is minimized. One could, indeed, make a case that the suffering the twins would endure in the NICU might exceed the harm of death. Forman, in recounting the various ethical complexities surrounding the birth of her preemies, acknowledges the suffering that they would face in the NICU, but her narrative does not mention a discussion of this possibility with her doctors.

Looking deeper into Forman's narrative, there is another possible reason why her desires for her twins were overridden. Within the confusion and disorientation of unexpected premature childbirth, she admitted that she did not think that she would be able to properly love and care for a disabled child and that she feared the changes in her own life that would result. In the first few days, she found herself thinking, *"Don't do this to me, don't change my life this way,"* so often that she calls it her "incantation" (p. 31). She also expressed these fears to medical staff. Perhaps the medical staff suspected Forman of following her own interests and did not fully trust her to make the proper decision for her babies.

However, Forman's right to make decisions for medical treatment for her babies, initially revoked, was oddly reinstated when it became clear that medical science was not up to saving the second twin. Once Ellie's death became inevitable, the doctors permitted Forman to make the decision to withdraw treatment, though many of them still objected. Ellie was removed from life support and allowed to die. But by then, Forman was beginning to adjust to her sudden motherhood. Her incantation of *"Don't do this to me"* had been coupled with *"Who will love them if not me?"* (p. 31). The four days that Ellie lived provided no reassurance to her mother. She says, "I will never have the answers to the questions surrounding Ellie and her short life. What if we hadn't insisted—would she have survived? What if we had been more ready to raise a profoundly disabled child—would that have made us better people?" (p. 31).

No one can answer those questions, and I do not wish to argue here the correctness of either the initial decision to resuscitate the twins or the later decision to withdraw aggressive care for Ellie. Ethical discussions of these topics abound in the neonatal literature surrounding resuscitation in the grey zone; the legal literature regarding the Baby Doe laws; and the ethics literature regarding children's best interests, parental rights, and the harm standard.

Nor do I wish to imply that Forman's experience is common. Despite literature showing that parents often do not fully understand the medical consequences of the decision to resuscitate (Keenan et al., 2005; Bastek et al., 2005; Boss et al., 2008) and that parents might feel pressured into accepting resuscitation (Harrison, 2008), I believe that most parents freely choose resuscitation. A survey of parents, including those of both full term and extremely premature infants, found that 64% of parents believed that attempts should be made to save all infants at birth, regardless of their condition (Streiner et al., 2001).

Instead, I want to briefly examine one way in which the decision altered the life of the twins' mother. Forman was quite honest in relating her worries about the effect that disabled twins might have on her life. The doctors questioned her reasons for refusing resuscitation and reframed the disagreement about whether life or death was in the twins' best interest as an inappropriate and possibly selfish attempt by their mother to avoid caring for them. When it became clear that Ellie would not survive, Forman had to fight to end her suffering. The emotional consequences of this are clear in her narrative. She was unable to process her grief. Ellie's ashes lived on the radiator in her parents' bedroom for fourteen months.

Jacqueline Slomka, an anthropologist and nurse who studied life-and-death decisions in the ICU, observed that medical staff decisions are often framed in a way that avoids personal responsibility for the limits of medicine and the reality of death. Death is avoided until every possible avenue for treatment has been tried in order to assure that no one can be held morally accountable for it (Slomka, 1992). By accepting the inevitable, and asking for death to be hastened, Forman took on full responsibility for Ellie's death, unsupported and unacknowledged. Essentially the blame for the failure of medicine to save Ellie was transferred to Forman, who then had to live with her decision. The burial of her daughter's ashes fourteen months later was merely the beginning of dealing with the guilt and doubt this engendered. She was still processing it on the final pages of her memoir.

But that dilemma pales in comparison to the ethical questions raised by the survival of the second twin. By far the most significant portion of her memoir deals with Forman's life with her surviving child. Evan lived for eight years in a state of near-total dependency. For most of that time, his mother was his primary caregiver. It is this portion of Forman's story which I believe deserves most of our attention. *This Lovely Life* describes the slow transition Forman made from reluctant parent to caregiver for a child with multiple, severe disabilities. It is the narrative of the new life that she took on when she became an extreme caregiver. It asks, but does not fully answer, several important questions: Can someone be a good mother after such a beginning? Was Evan's care too much to ask of her? Did Forman become, after desperately wanting him to die, a good caregiver for her son?

Evan's Story: A Narrative of Caregiving

Vicky Forman's surviving son, Evan, had a reasonably uncomplicated neonatal course, for a micro-preemie. However, the necessary ventilation caused minor lung damage, and the high oxygen damaged his eyes. A series of operations at three months of age failed to save his vision. Following the surgeries, his progress in feeding and developing slowed. At each setback, Forman feared she would be unable to handle a child with such problems, then learned very slowly to accept the new gap between her idea of normal and Evan's potential outcome. She learned even more slowly to trust in her abilities to care for him.

Evan was finally sent home at nearly six months of age with home oxygen, an apnea monitor, a gastrostomy tube, five medications, overnight continuous feedings, and follow-up appointments with six different specialists. He was blind, unable to take a full feeding from a bottle, and had yet to lift his head or smile.

During the six-month hospital stay, Forman states that she continued to distance herself from her son. She was afraid that he might die and wanted to protect herself from grief. Yet she stayed by his bedside, day after day, witnessing both the suffering of setbacks, major and minor, and the triumph of tiny steps toward discharge. When Evan came home, Forman finally felt that he would survive and that it was safe to love him. She says, "In coming home, I surprised myself. I fell in love with my son" (p. 146).

She also began a round of caregiving that was more taxing than the prolonged hospitalization had been. The book documents the schedule for feeding and medications, and the observation from Evan's grandparents that they seemingly had brought the NICU home with them. Within a few weeks, Forman discontinued the apnea monitor, because of the frequent, useless false alarms that disrupted the little sleep she was able to get. This did nothing to improve the relationship between Forman and Evan's doctors, already eroded by the knowledge that she had not wanted the twins resuscitated.

And Evan's setbacks were not over either. At follow-up visits he was diagnosed with a life-limiting defect in one of his heart valves and, later, low-tone cerebral palsy. Both of these diagnoses were pronounced with a callousness that caused Forman initially to deny their existence and insist, to herself and others, that her son was not disabled. At nine months old, Evan began having seizures which were initially trivialized by his doctors. In a reversal of her former denial, Forman fought for better treatment. It was by her own persistence and advocacy that Evan was seen by a pediatric neurologist who recognized the seizures as infantile spasms, a form of epilepsy which has a particularly poor prognosis.

Forman did not chronicle Evan's later years in detail, but by age five, he was off both oxygen and tube feedings. His seizures had mysteriously stopped. He was eating soft foods, drinking from a cup, and beginning to take a few steps. His mother had come to terms with Ellie's death, seeing it as a willing sacrifice for the life of her brother. She had become Evan's fearless supporter and advocate. Through caring for Evan, she had learned to accept and value her blind and severely disabled son.

His death was sudden and unexpected. She says, "We want, in an ending, a sense of justice and purpose, a feeling that the inexorable is also comprehensible. In truth, no ending is ever complete, no goodbye sufficient. I was not done with my son, and yet he died. Did that mean he was done with me?" (p. 258).

In that final, agonizing question lies a world of ethical dilemmas. At the end of her memoir, Forman still has no mechanism to understand the consequences, both for her son and herself, of Evan's premature birth and unprepared-for life. Like all of us, she does not know the answers to the existential question of why he lived or why he died. But she also has no measure by which she can determine whether she adequately fulfilled her role in his life as mother and caregiver. She is asking the reader if his death was a final judgment of her performance as an extreme caregiver; the ultimate in failure.

Forman was given the task of raising her severely disabled son, a task she did not want, and for which she was, because of her opposition to the

NICU, suspected of being inadequate. No one considered the enormous changes in her life and in herself with which she had to wrestle, alone and grieving, at Evan's bedside. No one noticed whether she felt safe to love him, or not. She took Evan home, in much the same way as she was assigned Ellie's death, unacknowledged and unsupported, because she was his mother. Even she wondered about her competence and adequacy for the task. Yet she became her son's principle caregiver, his best advocate, and his loving mother.

The complexity of Forman's narrative makes it clear that describing and defining the lives of extreme caregivers is essential, but it is merely a beginning. While it is certainly important to recognize the difficulty of the task that she, and parents like her, are doing, I believe it is imperative also to elucidate the moral work they must do. I think Forman did more than her moral duty; she did an exemplary job against enormous odds. But to explain why I think that, we need a different approach to ethics; a way to look at her narrative, and the narratives of other extreme caregivers, from new angles.

Other Methods of Ethical Analysis

The undeniable existence of children like Evan challenges the defined boundaries of medical care and of parenting. It also calls for expanding our understanding of ethics and the kinds of questions asked about children with multiple disabilities. We need to examine the process Forman went through in order to transform from mother into extreme caregiver. We need a way to evaluate whether, despite being in opposition to the medical community, Forman performed her caregiving tasks admirably. We need to understand the relationship between Forman and her son, not just while he was a patient in the NICU, but also once he came home into her care.

There is no established technique for ethically evaluating a narrative as complex as that offered by Forman and other extreme caregiving parents. So far, we have looked at Forman's story largely through the lens of Beauchamp and Childress's four principles, which is perhaps the most common way to look at the problems posed by Evan's birth. With their focus on autonomy and rights, Beauchamp and Childress's principles allow us to argue about what Evan's best interests might be and who should be empowered with their preservation. Once Evan was discharged from the NICU, Foreman was charged, by the fact of her motherhood, to provide the agreed-upon standard things that are owed to children: food, nurturing, and safety from bodily harm. The problems posed by Evan's survival—any difficulties that might arise in providing these things for a child with Evan's needs—were secondary to the requirement to meet them.

Feminist ethicist Margaret Urban Walker (1992) has described this model for ethical analysis as following a "theoretical-juridical" model of morality. Theoretical-juridical theories, like principle ethics, rely on establishing rules that will apply in all, or most, situations. They consider emotions unimportant, or even undesirable, and favor individual, rational thought (Callahan, 1988). They also, according to Walker, often assume that all people are independent and rational individuals, always capable of looking out for themselves. However, it is difficult to use a system of ethics that relies on rights and autonomous choice to consider a state of dependency. It is also difficult to evaluate care and caregiving, which is by its nature relational. To evaluate a state of extreme dependency requires an ethic that acknowledges and accepts the existence of dependency and seeks to understand people in their relationships with each other. We need methods that examine the act of caring itself; a system for isolating important components of caregiving in order to examine them.

Some ethicists are working out different methods for making moral judgments, which follow what Margaret Urban Walker calls an "expressive-collaborative" model. Expressive-collaborative theories are based on relationships and emotions that previously went unnoticed. They depart from statements about autonomy and rights, and concentrate instead on community and interdependence, and the possibility of caring for each other (Walker, 1992). Some of those methods expand on an older form of ethics, virtue ethics, which was famously used by Aristotle, and examines morality through the development of character. The new expressive-collaborative model is one form of feminist ethics, all of which look primarily at the distribution of power and responsibility. Care ethics, also a feminist ethic, examines caring and the caregiving relationship.

In the field of medicine, where the stated focus is on providing care, an ethic based on care and caring seems an ideal match. Particularly when analyzing caregiving, as I intend to do, a system that acknowledges dependency and examines the caring relationship seems appropriate. It may not provide many (or better) answers, but the questions that emerge are very different from those often posed using rules and principles.

One expressive-collaborative model for better understanding and analyzing care was proposed by feminist ethicist and political scientist, Joan Tronto. In her book *Moral Boundaries: A Political Argument for an Ethic of Care* (1993), Tronto has outlined a way to understand care as a moral act done to fulfill a need. She has broken the act of giving care into four phases, each of which move an actor (either a person or group of people) closer to participating in the work of meeting needs. For each phase, she has proposed a virtue that can be used to ethically evaluate action in that phase. Tronto's proposed virtues can be used as a framework to spotlight the many activities, both physical and emotional, in which caregiving parents must engage in order to meet the complex needs of their children.

Some theories of care have been criticized for relying too much on the analysis of unreliable and unmeasurable emotions such as caring, empathy (Slote, 2007), compassion, or pity (Boyd, 2004). But, while caring is indeed an emotion that, for example, parents feel toward their children, the provision of care is an ongoing and active project which does not necessarily require the emotion called caring. Tronto's theories are based largely on the ability to recognize and meet needs. Unlike theories based on emotion, the recognition of needs and the successful meeting of those needs are measurable and actionable. Within that system, each phase of care holds a unique moral property or virtue on which to base action. These phases serve to separate the action of caring from the emotion called caring (or empathy or pity) and allow moral evaluation of the work done in each phase.

The focus on the identification and meeting of needs has the potential to turn the discussion of an ethic of care away from a somewhat vague and controversial analysis of the emotions of caring and toward an ethic where care becomes a politically actionable concept. Thus caring goes beyond a description of an emotion and instead encompasses reaching out to another and taking some action. Tronto recognizes that the action of providing care involves physical work, saying, "to care implies more than simply a passing interest or fancy but instead the acceptance of some form of burden" (1993, p. 103). Using Tronto's four phases of care and their associated virtues, we can leave behind the question of Forman's conflicted emotions toward her twins and instead consider what sort of burden she took up and whether she carried it well.

I have chosen the framework provided by Joan Tronto's phases of care to break down the complex and intense act of extreme caregiving into specific components, each of which can then be evaluated on both an emotional and morally actionable level. To do this, I must expand Tronto's theories, perhaps in ways she never intended. Since I rely on concepts developed from these four phases to provide a framework to analyze caregiving narratives, it is necessary to review this part of Tronto's theories.

I summarize them here, then review each phase and its associated virtue in more detail separately.

Tronto's four phases of caring are, briefly: (1) Caring about. This is the closest to the emotion of caring, as it involves the usually empathic awareness that someone is in trouble. However, Tronto's definition requires only being open to the world and being willing to notice unmet needs. (2) Taking care of. This involves taking on some of the work of care, agreeing to help meet a need, but in an indirect manner. Things like making a contribution to a disaster relief fund, working for a day at Feed My Starving Children, or becoming an activist for people with disabilities are all ways to indirectly take care of a need. (3) Care-giving. The caregiver is the heart of caring, doing the often unrecognized dirty work of care. Caregiving is direct action: cleaning the muck out of flooded houses, preparing and delivering meals, or actually helping build necessary wheelchair ramps. In health care, it is the changing of bedpans, the holding of hands, the coming in response to a distress call. This phase involves doing the direct, hands-on work of care. Thus care is a practice, an action that can be learned, not an emotion or a principle (Tronto, 1993, pp. 105–108).

The last phase is: (4) Care-receiving. In this phase, the caregiver double-checks the adequacy of the care that has been performed. This is an interesting and somewhat different phase, because it requires participation from the cared-for. It also calls upon the participants in the first two phases—those who notice and support the fulfillment of needs—to ensure that the needs of the caregiver are also being adequately met.

To each of her four phases of care, Tronto has assigned an associated virtue that guides us in how to act in each of those degrees of closeness to care. The virtue associated with "caring about" is attentiveness. A person who demonstrates this will stay open to the recognition of needs of others and likely will find many. They may feel sympathy or pity, but it is not a necessity. The virtue needed for the second phase, "taking care of" is responsibility (or taking responsibility) and is a call not merely to notice needs but also to be ready to take some personal stake in meeting them. For the third phase, the caregiver must be able to perform care that meets the needs that are present, so the virtue required for caregiving is competence in the provision of care. This emphasizes that learning how to do care work properly is an important part of the process of caring. Tronto has assigned to the fourth phase of care, care-receiving, the virtue of responsiveness. She means this to be a virtue exercised by the caregiver, who must nurture a relationship with the care-receiver, which, at the very least, must include eliciting a response from the care-receiver regarding the effectiveness of the care.

The virtues that Tronto has assigned to the phases of care are modeled after Aristotelian virtues, where moral behavior is understood to be a mean between two extremes. A virtue can be thought of as a sort of middle ground for behavior, which is surrounded by less desirable actions or attitudes of the same sort. Aristotle explores the quality of moral virtues by identifying associated extremes of undesirable (or less moral) behavior and attempting to find a moral balance. By assessing the dangers of their extremes, he is able to zero in on the best qualities behind various virtues. Tronto does not specify the sort of extremes to be avoided for each virtue of her phases of care, however, I will propose my own interpretation as I consider each phase individually.

I will also use a different, more modern, form of virtue ethics. Virtues can also be analyzed as commendable character traits that can be developed for moral improvement. This method of virtue ethics focuses on a range of available actions, takes emotions into account, and emphasizes the connection between the moral agent and the community of which he is a part. My favorite definition of virtues comes from a nursing ethics textbook, which states, "Virtues are complex, learned dispositions that enable individuals to perceive, feel, and act appropriately in response to the challenges and circumstances of their communal lives. Instead of focusing on rules to direct our responses, virtue ethics emphasizes the development of the ability to perceive, feel, and act appropriately in changing and complex circumstances" (Volbrecht, 2002, p. 99). With this definition in mind, we can also examine the ways in which Tronto's phases and their virtues direct the actions of caregiving and link action with character development that will, perhaps, provide moral direction for that action. However, when considering virtues as guidance for character development, caring-as-action cannot be entirely separated from caring-as-emotion. Indeed, some of the moral work that must be done by caregivers involves coming to terms with emotions.

In much of the analysis of work in health care, specifically nursing, that follows Tronto's phases, including in some of her own work, all four phases of care are assigned to the individual nurse caregiver. Thus a nurse is called upon to care about and to take care of; to be attentive and responsible. She, of course, must be competent in her caregiving duties. In addition, she must be responsive to the care-receiver's needs, even if her patient is not in a position to provide consistent verbal feedback.

I will also use the concepts of attentiveness, responsibility, competence, and responsiveness mostly on an individual level, but I must stress that this is not the only way they can be used. The four phases are much more versatile than personal virtues and can also be applied at a societal or political level, as well as to the work of a single nurse or caregiver. The phases, applied to a medical system, are not merely stages which a single actor or potential caregiver goes through as she approaches the need for care. They are degrees to which any agent or agency is involved in the caring process: from recognition of a need through accomplishing the hard work of meeting it. In a wider system, attentiveness and responsibility enacted by others, both toward the care-receiver and the caregiver, would likely improve the final result. Competence and responsiveness on the part of any agency delivering health care would also likely promote the fair recognition and efficient meeting of needs.

The four phases of care acknowledge that all of us are interdependent and rely on others for some sort of care. Those who do not recognize their need for care are likely failing to notice important ways in which their lives are being maintained by others, through underappreciated tasks such as housekeeping, maintenance, and services. It also acknowledges that, at some point, any of us could find our need for care increasing and become the care-receiver of a different or more intense level of care.

More recently, in her book *Caring Democracy*, Tronto (2013) has described a fifth phase of care, which she calls "caring with." In this phase, the participants in a society, particularly a democracy, engage in practices that support and encourage caring behavior. Currently, care is relegated to the private sphere and is something that we all must arrange for individually. Tronto proposes that consideration of the care we all require should be central in the public sphere. She states, "Unless democrats, as people committed to both equality and freedom, are willing to offer an alternative account of how we might care, then . . . caring [will continue to be viewed merely as] a choice one makes about how to exercise one's personal responsibility" (p. 44). I agree that public policy shaped to best meet the needs of all would be desirable. However, this phase does not directly apply to caregiving by individual parents, so I did not use it in my analysis of parent narratives. I believe that once the extent of extreme caregiving becomes apparent, some "alternative account of how we might care" will be necessary. We return to this phase in the final chapter, where I discuss possible actions to take to relieve parent caregivers.

I believe that when we examine the work of parent extreme caregivers by using Tronto's phases to pinpoint aspects of the task, we will be able to break down this complex task into comprehensible components. We will be able to determine where extreme caregiving differs from typical parenting merely by the level of complexity, and where its intense nature becomes morally problematic. I hope also that this will teach us something about the nature of caregiving itself. As the difficulty and consequences of extreme caregiving become clear, I believe that the need for others in the health care system to take action in some of the phases of care will be obvious.

Caring About

"Caring about" is the first phase of caring, and, seemingly, the phase that requires the least amount of personal involvement. It is also the phase that seems closest to an emotion. The phrase, caring about, is frequently used to describe emotional involvement. I have said that some theories of care have been criticized for being too reliant on emotions, and so I must point out the ways in which caring about and its associated virtue, attentiveness, are similar to, and differ from, the emotions of caring, pity, and empathy.

We are all capable of caring about those who are close to us. Caring about strangers is more difficult, but certainly possible, though we often require that their need be waved in our faces before we recognize it. But the virtue of attentiveness is a quality that implies a certain way to look at the world, not a way to feel about others. It demands that one notices the needs of others and recognizes both the possibility of fulfilling them and those who are already doing that work.

The emotions of caring have been criticized for their potential to become too personal, too likely to result in unfair advantages to those we hold dear, or who happen to be in range of our vision. This can lead to an unequal distribution of care, as only the needs of those we already care about are noticed. Insufficient attentiveness can also lead to a sort of paternalism, where the focus narrows in on certain needs and ignores others that may be of more importance.

Ethicist Steve Edwards has stated that one of the advantages of Tronto's phases is that they can be applied impartially and that this impartiality is an "essential element" of any ethical system (2009, p. 233). "Caring about" which is directed by impartial attentiveness, can be expressed in a way that turns caring into an action that can be applied with justice in mind, not merely an emotion that will only be aroused unreliably. I suspect that complete fairness is not essential (or attainable), but an ethical system must have some measure of impartiality to be useful.

Caring as an emotion and attentiveness when giving care are both subject to the possibility of over-involvement. While too little attentiveness will express itself in self-interest and a scattered and unreliable recognition of the need for care, excess attentiveness could potentially lead to the loss of selfhood in the caregiver. The caregiver can become so focused on the needs of another that her own desires and life goals are put aside.

Indeed, some feminist philosophers have critiqued the idea that caregivers should be selfless, as sometimes expected in the past. They state that it is not necessary for the caregiver to put aside her own ego and personal interests in order to give good care (Bowden, 1998, p. 61). This depth of attentiveness toward others can lead to an emotional, and possibly ecstatic, engrossment in the other, which can be a source of joy. But it can also lead to a loss of one's selfhood—a self-abrogation or denial that could ultimately be self-destructive. Philosopher Peta Bowden (1998) points out that this self-erasure is all too close to the disenfranchising self-denial that, historically, women as default caregivers must overcome. Applied to an ethic of care, this could lead caregivers to define their selves and desires almost entirely in terms of the interests of others.

Many feminist philosophers, including Bowden, agree that ethical attentiveness to another, if not taken to extremes, will ultimately lead to a broader self-understanding. The action of attentiveness might lead to the creation of a worldview that notices and values others, and then cycles back toward self-enrichment. This is an ongoing process that requires intelligence, imagination, and possibly education about the world inhabited by the other. Bowden states, "[N]ot only does attentiveness directed to others reflect back on oneself in enriched possibilities for self-knowledge, but that correspondingly, ethical attentiveness to oneself, one's limits and prejudices, facilitates revised and augmented possibilities for attention to others" (1998, p. 72). Thus proper attention leads to personal growth in both the subject of the attention and the attentive person. What emerges is an ideal of attention as an act of looking clearly at another with a sort of patient expectancy, waiting to understand who they are and what their needs might be.

Though Bowden is not specifically talking about caring for children, parents of both sick and well children must apply ethical attentiveness in parenting. An attitude of patient expectancy, and waiting to understand who a child is and what her needs might be, may well define excellent parenting. It is certainly possible for parents to be attentive in a way that both engrosses and enriches them, without causing them to lose their selfhood. However, both extremes of inattentiveness and over-attentiveness exist in parenting, with children harmed by neglectful or suffocating parents, and parents submerging both too little and too much of themselves in their children. For parents of children with multiple health care needs, however, attentiveness must unavoidably be set at a high level, threatening the parent's sense of selfhood.

One of the many things to which Forman was supposed to be attentive was an apnea monitor. Her memoir does not report the type of monitor, nor the indications for its use, but only the confession that she discontinued it against medical advice. At the time, monitors were routinely prescribed to NICU graduates on a preventive, "just in case" basis. I prescribed many of them. Many parents found them comforting, at least initially. However, the monitor consisted of a foam band fastened around the baby's chest with velcro. The electrodes inside the band would lose contact with the baby's skin whenever the baby moved, causing a loud alarm. The parent, listening intently and fearfully for such alarms, would run panicking into the baby's room, to find nothing whatsoever wrong. After the first few times, the constant need for alertness, dulled by peaks of unnecessary panic, took its toll, causing many parents increased anxiety, guilt, and self-doubt. A dozen alarms per day were not unusual.

Since identifying virtues associated with care is an attempt to define moral behavior, this level of attentiveness seems to set a different moral standard for some parents. Vicky Forman seemed well aware of this, and for her the need for attentiveness became entangled with self-blame. Forman states,

> In the stories I read later of children dying and bereaved parents, there was always the sense of foreboding, of having made a mistake by allowing the night out, the boat trip on the lake, the ski weekend . . .. In the same way that a mother clings to details, she also believes that if she simply pays attention long and hard enough, she can prevent anything from happening. (2009, p. 54)

Perhaps, for Forman, the need for constant vigilance fed her fear that lack of attentiveness will result in tragedy or that tragedy must always be due to lack of attentiveness.

To analyze parent caregiving in its most difficult form, I must assume that parents of both typical and special needs children share an equal capacity to "care about," and that they will be attentive in very similar ways. Parents of medically complex children will find more needs to notice and pay attention to, but their ability to recognize those needs is not usually in question. Instead, in this phase, we must analyze the emotional result that might be produced by an increased and prolonged need for attentiveness, and the moral work that must be done to maintain that level of awareness.

Taking Care Of

The next question in Tronto's ethic of care is how to direct that hard-won moral attention. The mere knowledge of need is only a small step toward meeting that need. The second of Tronto's phases of care is "taking care of," which Tronto defines as being willing to take some action toward meeting a need that has been noticed. She has assigned to it the virtue of responsibility (Tronto, 1993). To analyze this, we need to know the extent to which the recognition of a need obligates a response to that need. We need to think about what it means to take on responsibility.

Philosopher John Caputo, in his essay "Against Ethics," recognizes that needs, when noticed, will sometimes evoke a response, which he identifies as obligation. The recognition of a present need sometimes calls forth an urgent and sympathetic desire to help. He defines obligation as "the feeling that comes over us when others need our help, when they call out for help, or support, or freedom, or whatever they need, a feeling that grows in strength directly in proportion to the desperateness of the situation of the other" (1993, p. 5). However, in the context of caregiving, the form that response should take is not clear. Caputo states that obligation often comes unexpectedly and chaotically. But there is no good answer to the question of which needs, when noticed, call forth an obligation or a requirement to act.

It seems to me that responsibility as a virtuous act might be the deliberate acknowledgment or acceptance of Caputo's obligation. Recognizing a need, we act, not from some assigned duty or in response to the rights of the vulnerable, but because we agree to take responsibility for some part of the necessary care. In doing so, I believe we often must willingly sacrifice some degree of our independence in order to attend to the needs of others.

It is possible to consider the virtue of responsibility as a mean between extremes; however, it is perhaps easier to recognize a lack of responsibility than it is to imagine an overabundance of it. Though it is certainly possible for someone to take on more problems than they can handle, we are more likely to identify a moral wrong if someone ignores needs that should be their responsibility. It is also not clear to me exactly how those extremes might be avoided, particularly by parents who have taken on the responsibility for raising a child and find the job more difficult than they expected.

Rather than assigning blame to parents who take on too little or too much responsibility, it may be more useful to examine the sorts of responsibilities that come with parenting and consider ways to relieve those who find themselves overburdened.

It seems to me that an ethic of responsibility might be impossible within a society that, like ours, is not focused on recognizing and meeting each other's needs. There is no process by which responsibilities that have been taken on, but can't be met, can be passed to another person. There is not even a process by which extra burdens can be recognized. The first step toward relieving the additional burdens that come with extreme caregiving, then, is to identify the extra responsibilities parents have been given.

Accepting responsibility for raising a child is a clear obligation of parenthood. Parents are judged on their ability to take on a variety of responsibilities, and parenting books are filled with advice on how to meet them. Most parents understand that this is a part of the parenting process. Vicki Forman has no doubts of this. She says, of her multiply disabled son, "No matter what, I am his mother and it is and will be my job to take care of him" (2009, p. 109). The parents of children with special health care needs do not differ from the parents of typical children in this acceptance, but there is no ethic to dictate the circumstances under which they might be permitted to put some of their extra responsibilities aside.

I have said that Forman, when she asked for the withdrawal of aggressive treatment for her daughter, took responsibility for Ellie's death. This is not something parents are usually asked to do. While some might view this as an immoral and irresponsible act, many neonatologists and ICU physicians are beginning to believe that aggressive treatment in the face of immanent death is inappropriate because it often merely prolongs suffering. Forman chose to face her daughter's death immediately, rather than watch her die slowly over days. In this view, she did not shirk her responsibility to care for Ellie by promoting her death, but instead she took on an enormous burden of responsibility. That this decision became her sole responsibility, with only minimal support from the medical team, then can be seen as an unfair assignment of responsibility.

Forman suggests that some of that responsibility for caring for children with special needs who survive also belongs to the medical system and that the system is not doing a very good job of it. After Evan's discharge from the hospital, she did not receive the help she needed. She says, "If the doctors had lined up at Evan and Ellie's birth to do the impossible, to prove all that medical science could do to save one-pound babies, I was to learn how little those medical professionals on the other side of that accomplishment could or would do to help" (p. 167). It is true that Forman's relationship with her son's medical team was unusually contentious. However, I agree that Evan and Ellie's neonatologists, by the intense nature and complexity of the care they gave, do indeed hold some responsibilities toward the twins' future beyond the NICU. And I believe that it is likely, since we are lacking a complete understanding of the responsibilities that fall on extreme caregiving parents, that the medical system is not adequately performing all of its responsibilities.

In Chapter 5 I consider both of the first two phases of care together. The ethical and emotional consequences of the two phases are similar and, at times, overlap in a way that makes it impossible to separate them. Parents of children with multiply disabilities or intellectual delays must exercise acute attentiveness in multiple areas and are obliged to take on numerous and difficult responsibilities. We shall see that the cost of this hyper-awareness and over-obligation is high. I believe also that the difficulties encountered by extreme caregiver parents, once made visible, should in turn call forth an obligation from all of us as members of a moral community.

Care-giving

Caregiving is the heart of caring, an action both under-recognized and absolutely necessary. Tronto has assigned the virtue of competence to the hands-on caregiver. The reason for this is fairly simple: care given incompetently does not meet the need and therefore is inadequate (Tronto, 1993). As we shall see, the emotion of caring or empathy is not required for the action of caregiving, although it may be desirable and at times necessary for doing it well. In some forms of caregiving, I suspect emotion is unavoidable.

Competence as a virtue is most understandable when considering the physical act of caregiving. For the work of caring, in health care as in other fields, you want people who do it well. For a sick patient in the hospital, you want people who know how to change bed linens without causing pain, how to work the suction equipment, how to start an IV. You want people who know what lab tests to order, are good at obtaining them, and know what they mean. You want nurses and doctors who have passed their boards, who aren't working while impaired, who are competent. All of this can be done, and perhaps even done well, without any emotional attachment.

Defining professional competence is not terribly difficult. A performance within certain scientific standards is expected, and measurements of competence have already been applied to the practices of medicine and nursing. Defining competence as a virtue balanced between extremes, however, is not terribly useful. Rather than attempting to determine a morally desirable level of competence, it might be more important to define the tasks at which a caregiver should excel. The areas of competence we consider desirable, and what sort of training we expect in a caregiver, will determine the kind of care we receive.

Most of us are aware that competence in the form of scientific prowess does not, by itself, ensure good health care. Care focused only on tests and standards, for example, might fail to take into account the whole patient, particularly the way in which the patient experiences illness. You also want nurses and doctors to do only what is necessary; that is, not ordering excessive tests or performing unnecessary procedures. Following a technological imperative to do things because they are available or are reimbursed well or will result in a great research paper is not evidence of competence.

Some have suggested that the harshness of technical competence can be abated by bringing emotions, particularly compassion or empathy, back into the picture. Nursing ethicist Berit Lindahl, for example, states, "Competence without compassion can be brutal and inhuman, and the reverse, compassion without competence, is meaningless or, at worst, dangerous" (Lindahl et al., 2006, p. 897). I agree, but requiring compassion from the caregiver returns us to relying on the presence and strength of an emotion in order to evaluate care. Tronto has not overlooked the possibility of care becoming paternalistic or harsh, however. We shall see how care can be moderated by relying on feedback from the care-receiver in the fourth phase of care.

We cannot leave emotion entirely behind, however. The moral caregiver, acting competently, must develop Volbrecht's "ability to perceive, feel, and act appropriately" in the changing environment of health care (2002, p. 99). Competence executed well must encompass emotional development, as well as technical prowess. The type of training received by health care providers determines which actions are considered important and appropriate in the delivery of care.

The focus here is not on the virtues of medical providers but on the family caregiver, however. Family caregivers are indeed required to gain some scientific knowledge, so it is important to examine how they approach that knowledge. It is likely also that they have something to teach medical providers about the emotional components of caregiving, but in evaluating extreme caregiving parents, compassion toward their children is not usually in question. For now, I think it is more important to look at the sorts of tasks that we have asked parents to do and the ways in which they become adept at them.

There are no standard requirements for competence in the caregiving task that is parenting, but the task is fairly well defined, and its success can be measured somewhat by the physical and emotional growth of the child. Likewise, there are few recognized standards for competence in caring for a medically complex child at home. A standard for competence in extreme caregiving, particularly for a child with intellectual disabilities, is even harder to find. With each child on an uncharted and sometimes completely unknown developmental path, there are few established milestones, and no definition for measuring success.

In caring for a child with special health care needs, we shall see, competence is often defined by the ability of the parent to provide medical and nursing care. This expectation often begins in the hospital, with parents scrambling to understand their child's medical problems. Prior to discharge from the hospital, parents must acquire a set of nursing skills that have been defined by their doctors using guidelines provided by the American Academy of Pediatrics (AAP) (Elias & Murphy, 2012). Many feel that these are inadequate, and parents report feeling unprepared and uncomfortable with medical caregiving for months following discharge (Ray, 2002). The level of preparation required can be astonishingly high.

Vicky Forman (2009) acquired competence slowly, as her son's setbacks required changing levels of care. When Evan was finally sent home from the hospital, he took his "own little ICU" (p. 140) with him in the form of "fifteen diagnoses, nine-page discharge summary, oxygen, feeding pump, and monitor" (p. 136). The amount of information required was overwhelming, and Forman states that the first few months "were a blur of responsibilities and phone calls and chores" (p.139). In addition to learning to use a GT-tube and administer medications, she used the internet to inform herself about all of her son's many complications. But the hardest task was coming to terms with her new duties, a much more complicated process. She had to learn a new way of life, and a new set of expectations, for both her own life and her son's. Among the many things she learned was a knack for knowing when to refuse medical advice.

Becoming competent required developing a combination of coping skills and acceptance. After confirming a new diagnosis of infantile spasms, a pediatric neurologist asks Forman how she is doing, and she says she is "okay." She writes, "That one question, amid all the hard news

I'd just heard, was enough to make me, at that moment, some new version of okay, one where *okay* meant *I can take this, I can do this, I can walk out of here with all this news and figure out how to go on.*" (p. 186) In this new world, becoming competent means more than acquiring nursing skills.

There is no precedent for requiring, acquiring, or maintaining the level of expertise these parents must achieve, practically and emotionally. The implication in guidelines, such as those provided by the AAP, is that competence can be gained easily by any parent, as long as they are given the right sort of training. Yet the extent of caregiving these parents are expected to carry out is much greater than such guidelines recognize. The guidelines also imply that technical competence is all that is needed, and that learning to live with a new definition of OK, as Forman did, requires neither skill nor effort.

The only people completely aware of the level and types of competence needed to carry out extreme caregiving, I believe, are the parents who are doing it. In Chapter 6, I discuss the variety of tasks in which extreme caregivers are expected to acquire competence, and the ways in which they acquire and frame that competence. I will examine the ways in which parents think about their own competence, and compare it with their impressions of professional competence. This information might be useful not only when preparing nonprofessionals to care for their children with special health care needs at home but also to increase our understanding of the important task of family caregiving.

Care-Receiving

Tronto (1993) called the fourth phase in her phases of care "care-receiving" and assigned to it the virtue of responsiveness. In this phase, the caregiver initiates a response from the person being cared for, regarding the acceptability and appropriateness of the care given. Typically the care-recipient is in the best position to determine what his needs are, and if those needs are being adequately met in the care that has been received. Ideally, this phase creates a feedback loop in which care is given, a response to the care is provided, and care altered accordingly.

This interaction also ensures that the recipient of care is not merely a blank slate on which care is written. Care ethicists recognize, as does Tronto, that "[t]o be in a situation where one needs care is to be in a position of some vulnerability" (1993, p. 134). The vulnerable care-receivers face "dangers . . . at the hands of their care givers and other champions, who may come to assume that they can define the needs of the vulnerable"

(p. 135). The cycle of responsiveness ensures that care is offered, rather than imposed, and is meant to, in some part, reduce the vulnerability of the care-receiver to the caregiver. The feedback of responsiveness ensures that the care given is actually necessary and desired by the care recipient. In this way, care will not be provided merely because a caregiver thinks it is needed, and care will not be paternalistically imposed on an unwilling and vulnerable recipient.

In addition, assigning responsiveness as a virtue emphasizes the relational nature of care. Few disagree that this relational component is an essential part of care, and some even argue that care not responded to is not truly caring. Feminist philosopher Nel Noddings believes that care provided is incomplete unless there is a response to it. She uses the word "reciprocity" to describe something very like responsiveness. Stressing that the giving of care is essentially a relationship, Noddings states that caring depends on reciprocity between caregiver and cared-for. She states, "As we examine what it means to care and to be cared for, we shall see that both parties contribute to the relation; my caring must be somehow completed in the other if the relation is to be described as caring" (1984, p. 4). The reciprocal relationship between caregiver and cared-for is essential and completes the caring process.

Tronto's virtue of responsiveness differs slightly from reciprocity in that it is possible to interpret it as an action, a direct inquiry into the state of care from caregiver to care-receiver that does not necessarily require the emotion of caring. But holding responsiveness as a virtue seems to me to require more than a mere checklist monitoring of care effectiveness. It also requires building a relationship. This raises the question of exactly what sort of responsive or reciprocal relationship is required for caring to be considered complete.

The first problem that arises here is that the ability of the care-receiver to participate in the relationship cannot be entirely controlled by the caregiver. If care must be responded to in order to be complete, it would be impossible to properly care for someone who is unable to respond at all, as in a persistent vegetative state. Clearly that is not the case. Caring for a person with dementia or intellectual disability, or even for a preverbal child, will hold different challenges. And there are also ways in which the care-receiver can undermine and make unpleasant the caregivers' tasks, thus complicating their own need for care.

By identifying the fourth stage of care as "care-receiving" Tronto meant to bring both caregiver and care-receiver into the care equation. Certainly the virtue of responsiveness calls forth an action from the caregiver, but it can also be considered as an attribute of the person receiving care. The implication is that the care-receiver also has responsibilities in the relationship. Assigning a virtue to the care-receiver would in turn suggest that receiving care is a skill that might be mastered or an action that can be done morally. I believe that a state of vulnerability cannot negate the ability, or completely forgive the necessity, to act morally. Some infractions could constitute a moral wrong that cannot be excused by the vulnerability that is inherent in the need for care.

Evaluating the moral responsibilities of the care-receiver is outside the scope of this book, particularly since we will be largely considering care of children, who would not ordinarily be expected to provide a coherent response to care. But I do want to point out that the caregiver cannot be held entirely responsible for creating a reciprocal care-completing relationship. In situations where the care-receiver cannot be or is reluctant to be responsive, we can expect that the caregiver will try to elicit a response. In care situations in which the care-receiver is unable to respond, perhaps it is enough to remain open to a response. Tronto states, "The moral precept of responsiveness requires that we remain alert to the possibilities for abuse that arise with vulnerability" (1993, p. 135). It is possible to imagine a position so vulnerable that there is no ability to protest inadequate or unwanted care. Those protests will be heard only if the caregiver is willing to listen for them. It is clear that responsiveness as a virtue, in this case, must be upheld almost entirely by the caregiver.

The other, and more significant, problem with envisioning the fourth phase of care as a responsive and possibly emotional relationship is that there are different levels of emotional engagement appropriate for different types of caregivers. Completing the caring process by establishing a reciprocal or responsive relationship will vary greatly along the spectrum from professional health care provider to family caregiver.

If we consider the bioethical work that has been done in empathy and detachment in professional caregiving as an evaluation of responsiveness, the virtue of responsiveness is not completely unexplored territory. It is clear that an inability on the part of a health care provider to elicit an adequate response to care might impede the entire caregiving process. I will provide a brief exploration of responsiveness in professional care relationships before embarking on the even less explored area of family caregiving. I believe that for family and some long-term caregivers, where emotional detachment cannot be expected, a different type or amount of responsiveness would be expected.

For professional caregivers, too little responsiveness will result in a sort of hard-heartedness, where patients are treated as interchangeable bodies harboring interesting diseases. Too much responsiveness in health care providers is difficult to imagine, however, unless it results in a level of emotional investment that would interfere with the ability to provide competent medical or nursing care. Responsiveness in caregiving might fall somewhere between detachment and over-involvement.

Evaluation of professional health care in the absence of empathy or responsiveness is gaining importance. Noddings provides a description of care that is not caring, which is perhaps all too fitting of the callous way in which care can be delivered if there is no reciprocity or responsiveness between caregiver and patient:

> As we convert what we have received from the other into a problem, something to be solved, we move away from the other. We clean up his reality, strip it of complex and bothersome qualities, in order to think it. The other's reality becomes data, stuff to be analyzed, studied, interpreted. All this is to be expected and is entirely appropriate, provided that we see the essential turning points and move back to the concrete and the personal . . . . If I do not turn away from my abstractions, I lose the one cared-for. Indeed, I lose myself as one-caring, for I now care about a problem instead of a person. (Noddings, 1984, p. 36)

Note that care delivered in this way is inadequate, but also the person attempting care is lost to the relationship and is no longer a true caregiver. Instead, Noddings recommends turning away from the image of the patient as a set of data, toward an emotional caring for a whole person. The responsiveness in Tronto's fourth phase can be seen as the recognition of this emotional turning point—moving back to consideration of the whole, which completes the process of caring.

Too often, in my experience, considering the whole patient is shorthand for taking a social history, usually a minimal inquiry into risk-taking behaviors such as smoking and drug use. Professional training in this area usually concentrates on the communication of information to patients, and its effectiveness is measured in patient compliance with instructions (Frank, 2002, p. 20). For example, in an article in a medical journal promoting empathy in physicians, a physician argues that opportunities to convey information are often missed because physicians do not recognize verbal cues from the patient, which he calls "potential empathic opportunity continuers" (Neuwirth, 1997, p. 606). The writer admits that there is no established way to train physicians to recognize and respond to these moments. He is quite convinced however that, if used properly, the patient will "feel understood" and thus more likely to be compliant. This does not seem to me to be true responsiveness, since it advances the goals of the physician without acknowledging that the patient's goals might be different.

The ideal of clinical detachment worsens this distancing effect. Those who step beyond the social history and attempt to feel what the patient is feeling or imagine themselves in the patient's situation are felt to be in danger of losing the objectivity necessary to the effective practice of medicine. Jane Macnaughton, a professor of medical humanities, warns of the "dangerous practice of empathy," saying that "full experience of mutuality or understanding is not possible" in the clinical setting (2009, p. 1940). Medical practitioners who try to employ empathy and claim to feel what the patient is feeling have no grounds on which to base that claim. They are in danger of a self-delusional misunderstanding of the very person they are attempting to relate to. Imagining what the other person might be feeling, without seeking understanding from that person, is also not responsiveness.

However, in the same essay, Macnaughton states that providers could have what she calls a "momentary mirroring of that patient's feelings." She concludes, "Doctors do not need to feel the distress of their patients themselves to do something about it. We may have a momentary mirroring of that patient's feeling within us, but what we maintain is sympathy (feeling for not with the patient) and the need to respond" (p. 1941). I agree that care providers do not have to empathically feel the patient's pain, but they do have to understand that pain might be present. The patient's feelings may be "mirrored" by a sympathetic realization that the patient is a fellow human being whose situation and their response to it might be different from the care provider's. "Feeling for not with the patient" could then become a form of openness or ethical attentiveness to the needs of a person. The exact nature of those needs might be clearer if the care provider merely asks about them, ensuring that any care provided is appropriate. If the relationship between professional caregiver and care-receiver sustains that cycle of responsiveness, evolving over time, moral caregiving can be accomplished.

For a family caregiver, or a provider of long-term home care, however, the phase of care-receiving is perhaps more demanding. The emotional attachments that already exist, or emerge after a time of intimate caregiving, can both impede and enhance the process. The ongoing, reciprocal relationship between caregiver and cared-for will create emotional ties that must impact the responsiveness cycle. Indeed, it seems to me that the performance of caregiving will be so entwined with the process of responsiveness, and the emotions that result, that the moral caregiver might have difficulty *not* performing it.

Noddings has proposed that the family caregiver is likely to find personal reward in the constant cycle of needs satisfied. Parenting a small infant, for example, requires a constant, nonverbal interpretation of needs. The response to care, far from being elicited as a part of the caregiving process, seems to be almost instinctual. The feedback loop between parent and infant reinforces the relationship between them, often lightening the task of caregiving. As Noddings says, "I am also aided in meeting the burdens of caring by the reciprocal efforts of the cared-for. When my infant wriggles with delight as I bathe or feed him, I am aware of no burden but only a special delight of my own" (1984, p. 52).

Family caregivers, enmeshed in emotional attachments, are perhaps more likely to lose themselves in the care relationship. A life spent entirely responding to the needs of another is problematic, particularly if the cared-for is a child who cannot always express her needs. The caregiver might reach a level of emotional involvement or paralysis where good care becomes impossible. This level of emotional attachment could take the form of complete engrossment in the child. This is not only potentially damaging to the selfhood of the caregiver, who becomes lost in the other's needs, but may have consequences for the care-receiver as well.

The parent of a child with medical problems must constantly respond to the child's medical needs. Anthropologist Cheryl Mattingly recorded a story from the mother of a child with sickle cell anemia that demonstrates how being on the front lines of medical care can alter the relationship between parent and child. Sickle cell anemia often causes painful crises, which can become life-threatening. Young children often can't localize the pain, so any crying could be the first sign of a severe problem. The mother reported to Mattingly that she had learned to watch her daughter very closely for any sign of pain, ready to try to localize it and determine its severity. On the first day of summer camp, her daughter began crying inconsolably. The mother initially didn't understand her daughter's tears, because her first reaction was to look for pain. But her daughter was crying because she was scared of a new situation. The mother said, "Now most mothers would know that, right? Me? Because I'm just trying to figure out, well why is she crying? What's going on? Is she in pain? . . . So there's a lag, or a delay" (Mattingly, 2014, p. 111). Because of her extraordinary circumstances, she had trained herself to a particular sort of vigilance. The ordinary event, a child's loneliness or fear of leaving for camp without her mother, was overshadowed by medical concerns and became difficult to interpret.

Vicky Forman did at times reach what I feel was a worrisome level of responsiveness caring for her son Evan. As she gained more experience with his care, Forman became a marvelously attentive and responsive caregiver but seemed on several occasions in danger of losing herself. She describes an episode that emphasizes the depth to which the caregiving relationship between parent and child can go. She reports,

> My connection to Evan . . . eventually reached a point where I knew when a seizure was about to happen—I'd open his diaper and Evan would pee all over my hand and I'd think, *Here it comes*, and sure enough, he'd start to seize. Or I'd be in the front seat of the car and hear something off about his voice and I'd know, *He's having one* . . . .. In the world of seizures, many parents describe an aura that appears before the child is struck, a sense of something amiss that is nearly visible. I came to know this aura, just as eventually I could hear one of Evan's seizures even if I was in the other room—I'd just get it right away, I'd know, I'd be right there. (p. 191)

By this time in the narrative, Forman's son Evan is almost a year old and has been having the type of seizures called infantile spasms for several months. He has already failed several medications, including a semi-experimental one, and his mother has had time to adjust to the constant need to monitor his seizures.

Perhaps she has gone too far? She has clearly invested everything in her life toward Evan's care. She says, "The bonds of love, forged in the NICU and made even stronger in his homecoming, had grown ever tighter, so entrenched now as to become nearly visceral. This intensity left little room for anyone else. Only I was strong or daring or brave enough to go where Evan now went, to witness and become part of his haywire brain" (p. 190). The places Forman went with her son, her "journey with Evan" (p. 190), included, of course, taking him to doctor's offices and hospitals and tests. It also included, at one point, trying his medications herself, in an attempt to understand what was happening to him.

I do not believe that Forman's pharmaceutical experiment is common, but we will see that several other parents, in their memoirs, describe similar journeys with their disabled children. I have observed in practice a number of parents with a similar exquisite sensitivity to a child's needs, and researchers have reported other parents who share Forman's hypersensitivity to seizures (Ray, 2002). I will describe in Chapter 7 the way this extreme responsiveness is expressed and attempt to determine whether Forman's engrossment with her son, and other parents' similar actions, constitute desirable levels of responsiveness in caregiving, or an unforgiving and perhaps unavoidable over-involvement. Extreme caregiving parents, whose lives are lived almost totally as a response to their child's needs, likely have much to teach us about the difficulties and consequences of responsiveness.

The phases of care and their attendant virtues describe a sequence of caring actions that close into a cycle of care. All the phases call for some action, beginning with open attentiveness to needs, progressing to the acceptance of responsibility toward those needs, and then to skilled performance of the work that will fulfill those needs. The fourth phase completes the cycle of care, calling the caregiver into the action of eliciting a response from the cared-for. This action of responsiveness at the very least requires the caregiver to interact on a personal level with someone in need, responding to their emotional and physical needs. Caring is then a cycle of perceiving need, responding to that need, then resetting the perceived need in response to that response. It is a feedback loop, always in the process of being perfected.

I believe that one way to further an ethic of care is to determine how best to express the virtues in each phase of care and observe how they might translate into good (and moral) caregiving. I propose to do that through listening to narratives by the people who are performing the most extreme form of caregiving—parenting a child with multiple disabilities. These parents, whose lives become engulfed by their child's needs, are on the front lines of a move toward family caregiving, and there is an urgent need to understand the moral work they are doing.

CHAPTER 5 | Attentiveness and Responsibility
The Invisible Work of Care

JOAN TRONTO, IN establishing the four phases of care, assigned to each a virtue or actionable ethical component. So from the four phases of care—caring about, taking care of, caregiving, and care-receiving—come the "four ethical elements of care: attentiveness, responsibility, competence, and responsiveness" (Tronto, 1993, p. 127). Breaking down extreme caregiving into the four phases of care will, I hope, begin to elucidate both the nature and the moral consequences of this most difficult type of caregiving. This chapter begins to evaluate extreme caregiving in the first two, and least intimate, of Tronto's phases.

Like the earlier chapter on the work of caregiving, this chapter will correlate common themes from research interviews with stories from narratives. This will serve both to illuminate the problems encountered in raising children with special needs and show that the narratives I have chosen are not fiction. While the autobiographers were free as narrators to exaggerate or understate their problems, much of what they express is not outside the range of feelings or experiences reported by research on the families of technology-dependent children. This chapter will, however, advance into territory that has not been explored by researchers.

Some of the work being done in these two phases is common with typical parenting. I believe that parents of both typical and special needs children can be assumed to be equally able to enact the virtues of attentiveness and responsibility. Attentiveness, I have said, is maintaining openness to needs of others. Responsibility is beginning to take action that will meet those needs. Parenting seems to me to merge these two phases so that they are indistinguishable. The parent must focus on the needs of the child as part of the responsibility assumed in becoming a parent. The main difference in these two phases for extreme caregivers lies in the number of needs the extreme caregiver must be attentive to and take responsibility for, compared with the usual expectations of parenthood. The burden of care is larger, both in the amount of physical work required and in its emotional and psychological consequences.

I have discussed, in Chapter 3, some of the more obvious burdens of care: the enormous amount of physical work often required, the increased need for financial resources, and the isolating aspects of extreme caregiving. From this information, it is already possible to compile an introductory list of the extra responsibilities inherent in caring for a child with special needs. While likely no more attentive or responsible than parents of typical children, extreme caregiving parents have many more things to which they must be attentive and for which they must take responsibility.

Parents must translate the care prescribed by medical providers into the reality of their lives. Almost all must become adept at accessing the medical system and reading their child's individual signs of illness. They become not only caregivers but also care coordinators, case managers, advocates for their child's specific medical and educational needs, activists for the provision of special services, and secretaries in the complicated and time-consuming game of paperwork required by insurance and social services (Carnivale, 2006).

Those parents who require help in the home sometimes find themselves responsible for the finding, hiring, and training of their own home health care staff. They have to coordinate schedules, keep timesheets, and do the paperwork either to pay staff directly or arrange for payment (Ray, 2002). In addition, parents must seek out and make appointments for the multiple doctors and therapists usually involved. It is not unusual for a child to regularly visit several specialists—one for each separate medical problem—as well as a variety of therapists. Once the need for services becomes apparent, parents must seek out a provider and arrange for a means of payment. Every visit to a specialist or therapist comes with attendant insurance paperwork, often with additional forms or phone calls required to justify the treatment.

The last of the multiple unexpected parental responsibilities is that of educator. A federal mandate for appropriate education for all children does not mean that schools automatically adopt every new service, nor that they make it easy for parents to obtain the services they believe will best benefit their child. The required Individual Educational Plans (IEPs) are produced at the cost of long hours of meetings and are constantly in need of revision. It is not unusual for parents to have to visit the schoolroom regularly both to monitor the child's comfort in a new environment and to assist teachers with complicated care.

In the remainder of this chapter I explore several areas of responsibility that fall largely outside of the medical system. The first of these is living with an uncertain future, particularly when the child's health is fragile or when there are developmental or medical setbacks. This can produce both intense highs and lows, as well as unfounded feelings of guilt, all of which can be misinterpreted by acquaintances and medical practitioners alike. The second aspect is living with ambivalence. Some parents resent the caregiving burden while still taking pleasure in the lives they share with their children, which produces an ambivalence that should not be mistaken for unwillingness to perform caregiving or lack of love for their children.

The third area is a different and rarely explored type of advocacy. Certainly parents need to advocate for the child in many public arenas, from medical research to insurance coverage to education. But in addition many parents fight a more personal battle as they encounter stigma in daily life. Parents often encounter situations where they must unavoidably fight for acceptance for their child and themselves. Many of their responsibilities require fighting an ongoing battle to establish for the child a future in a society that does not seem to hold a place for him.

Lastly, many parents perceive a lack of choice in undertaking the task of caregiving, a sentiment which is easily misinterpreted in an age where selective abortion is becoming reality. Though parents are given an enormous burden with very little support, they are met with suspicion if they seem reluctant to take on the task. Asking for relief can be perceived as a sign of unwillingness or intolerance. The need for inclusion and acceptance of children with disabilities receives much attention from disability activists and academic communities but is rarely addressed from the perspective of the parent who is ultimately responsible for the life of the child.

Emotional Burden: Living with Uncertainty

A long time ago, when I was working as a pediatric intern in a major city, my team was called urgently to the emergency room, where a very sick child had just arrived by ambulance. Jeanette, as it turned out, was well-known to the hospital. My "boss" for the evening, a resident two years ahead of me in training, had been a witness to the successful resuscitation of Jeanette eighteen months earlier, one summer afternoon when she had been found face-down in a swimming pool, pulseless and unresponsive.

He had been a member of the team that had saved her, and then sent her home after weeks in the pediatric ICU. She survived with a heartbeat and spontaneous respirations, but very little else. She had been a healthy seven-year-old, but now she could no longer walk, or talk, or feed herself. She opened her eyes, but did not look at anything, and responded to nothing, not even to pain.

Her care at home must have been agonizing. She was back in diapers, and could no longer bathe herself or brush her own teeth. Instead of learning reading and writing, her schooling was a round of physical and occupational therapy. Despite physical therapy, her muscles had contracted, curling her thin body into a fetal position. She had a gastrostomy tube for feedings, but even slow feedings often refluxed up her esophagus into her airway causing her to choke. She spent much of her time in the hospital for feeding and respiratory problems. On arrival in the ER that night, she had a high fever and difficulty breathing, clear signs of aspiration pneumonia. She was on the verge of respiratory collapse.

The resident with me was near tears. He remembered the resuscitation all too well and seemingly still felt guilt for his role in snatching her back from death. Both of us, looking down at the ruin of a little girl, felt the call and appropriateness of that death. We considered the possibility of giving her parents the choice to let her go peacefully, this time.

We never asked. Her father came storming into the room, demanding loudly and angrily that we save her life immediately. I was struck by the fury of this response, and thought I saw under it a thick layer of guilt. Perhaps he'd been the one who was supposed to be watching her the day no one noticed when she fell into the pool. Or perhaps he resented the enormous caregiving burden that had been placed on his family. Or perhaps he'd secretly hoped for this very moment, a moment when he could let his daughter go, and now had to cover up this weakness with bluster.

I never found out what motivated Jeanette's father's outburst. It was so severe that he had to be removed from the room, and eventually the hospital, while we set to work. It was a good hospital, and we knew what we were doing. We dutifully saved Jeanette's life once again. I never shook the feeling that we, as practitioners of medicine, had become too good at saving lives. But, clearly the emotions with which I viewed Jeanette's continued existence were vastly different from her fathers'. Now that we have become even better at saving lives than we were thirty years ago, I believe we need to understand Jeanette's father, not just his anger and fear, but how that might be motivated by guilt or grief, and how overwhelming protectiveness and love might also play important roles.

In addition to the large physical burden, it is almost universally understood that caregiving for any disabled or chronically ill child carries a heavy emotional toll. According to the studies, the parents of technology-dependent children live in a state of constant vigilance, listening for alarms from equipment and monitoring for signs of serious illness. For the sickest children, fear of death or of finding their child dead is ever present (Kirk, 1998; Wang & Bernard, 2004; Carnevale et al., 2006; Cockett, 2012). For those who are not quite so fragile, parents worry about what the future will bring, particularly if the child will be dependent on their care long-term (Ray, 2002; Carnevale et al., 2006). These fears and worries contribute to chronic anxiety, sorrow, sleeplessness, high levels of stress, and depression (Wang & Bernard, 2004). Also present are frustration, anger, and guilt (Kirk, 1998).

Parents are also reported to be burdened with a great deal of emotional distress, including grief over their child's disabilities, sadness at the enormous difficulties their child must overcome, and sorrow over the loss of the child they were expecting. However, Sara Green (2007), a sociologist and mother of a daughter with severe cerebral palsy, reports that prolonged, severe emotional distress is actually fairly rare. She interviewed eighty-one mothers of children with disabilities and found that while care was "time consuming, expensive and physically exhausting," most of the mothers had moved beyond emotionally crippling grief (p. 155). Most of the mothers had found their sadness replaced by "the ability to love and cherish a child not in spite of or because of the disability but simply with it as an integral part of who he/she is" (p. 157). Those few who did experience continuing emotional distress were often further burdened by the societal perceptions that they should feel sad because of their child's limited prospects. For the most part however, Green asserts that parents are "tired, not sad" (p.151).

All of these emotions are evident throughout parent narratives, often running together in a tangled mix. All of the parents felt worry, fear, and anxiety, both while they were going through the process of diagnosis and once their fears were confirmed. There was a good deal of frustration and anger in this process as well; directed at the medical establishment's inability to provide an explanation or a cure, and at themselves for their own inability to save their children. All worried frequently about what their child's future would hold. Though few of their children were technology-dependent or medically fragile, and there was no need to listen for alarms or live in constant fear of death, there was no less need for vigilance. Some children must be monitored for escalating behavior outbursts, self-injury, toileting accidents, and hidden signs of the usual childhood illnesses. But the most frequent and complicated emotion was guilt, and it is here that the parents' narratives hold understanding that research does not. It is surprising just how many things the narrators felt guilty about.

Part of that guilt stemmed from imagined inadequacy in caregiving. Josh Greenfeld for example, found that he was somehow unable to perform much of the caregiving for Noah (1970). He alternately reported guilt, feeling a failure at fatherhood, resentment toward his wife and Noah, and admiration for his wife's caregiving abilities. Ian Brown (2011) and his wife, though they shared some duties, also frequently argued about how much responsibility each was taking. Several of the narrators had a second, typical child, and also expressed guilt about the time they spent on caregiving being taken away from the well sibling.

Some of the guilt was imposed from the outside, as scientific theories looked for insight into the nature of their child's disability. This was particularly true for Greenfeld and Charles Hart (1989), since their children were diagnosed with autism during a period of time when it was felt to be an emotional disturbance possibly brought about by poor parenting. As they progressed through a series of understandings about the diagnosis and cause of their sons' problems, they alternately accepted and rejected blame. When the Greenfelds learned about the theory that autism could be caused by maternal emotional detachment, for example, they both felt guilty because they had not wanted the pregnancy. But at other times, Greenfeld and his wife adopted other things to blame, taking turns at being the perceived guilty party; vitamin deficiency caused by diet, or a mild head injury that might have happened while the other was looking away. They even blamed genetics, arguing about whose genes were responsible for Noah's problems (Greenfeld, 1970, pp. 51–52). The nature of the guilt changed with the diagnosis under consideration.

Much of the guilt is unfounded. Ian Brown's son has a disorder with a clear genetic cause, which he could not possibly have controlled or prevented. No screening for it currently exists. Knowing this, Brown still expresses a surprising amount of guilt that stands against all the scientific evidence he collects about Walker's condition. He says, "Even a firm diagnosis cannot clear away the ancient sense of culpability that has been attributed to these random genetic events for literally thousands of years—the lingering swamp notion that there is always a reason such a disability occurs, that it is a punishment, and thus deserved" (Brown, 2011, pp. 122–123). I doubt that he is alone in that lingering, archaic feeling of being punished for some unknown crime, irrational though it might be.

In addition, parents express guilt over the failure of their child to progress. In the world of extreme caregiving, where there is no accepted measurement of success, parents have no way of reassuring themselves that they have done the best job possible. Brown is the most articulate about his inability to find a program that helps his son Walker. He speaks about the sadness, envy and guilt he feels when he inevitably compares his son to other children with the same syndrome, particularly if their children are less affected than Walker. Perhaps that other child's parents were better somehow; perhaps they were luckier, or more committed, or discovered some rare treatment that Brown did not, or implemented a new treatment in some earlier or more effective fashion. He reports, "Every parent of a compromised child knows this secret envy, mines its thick seam of guilt" (Brown, 2011, p. 125).

However, once the task of extreme caregiving is taken on, shouldering this guilt, along with other strong emotions, becomes an expected, if not fully embraced, part of life. Parents cannot live every day in guilt, sorrow, and grief. The many things that require attention become part of the daily routine. The responsibilities are, perhaps unknowingly, accepted. Ian Brown, in another passage from *The Boy in the Moon*, talks about the way in which Walker's care has become integrated into his life:

> Gradually, as the endless routine of caring for him and watching him and stopping him and stimulating him became familiar, my fear subsided, and my grief was transformed into an unusual loneliness. Life with him and life without him: both were unthinkable.
>
> As much as I tried to consider alternatives, I couldn't imagine not caring for him every day: couldn't imagine a day without the morning wake-up, the cleanup, the dressing, the school, the return home, the tired wailing, the sudden change and the bursts of sunny happiness, the feeding, the pointless teaching, the hilarity, the hospitals and doctors, the steady worry, the night rambles, all repeated every day until it ended, however that happened. (2011, p. 68)

Like the parents in Sara Green's study, Brown is not constantly consumed by guilt or sorrow. Walker's needs have become an accepted part of his life and, though the routine is time-consuming, it is not without moments of love and happiness. Brown might always be tired, but he is not always guilt-ridden or sad.

Josh Greenfeld has a similar recognition of his duties as caregiver. He writes, "We will do what we have to do. We will take care of him [Noah] as best we can until we can no longer take care of him. We will have him in our home and find ways to live in joy with him. And when we cannot enjoy him as much as I would like to, I will love him even more" (1970, p. 60). Like Brown, he balances the burden of caregiving against his enduring love for his son.

Parents everywhere find themselves making similar adaptations to the presence and needs of their children. Though the parents who are extreme caregivers have so many more needs to adapt to, they also have Brown's "bursts of sunny happiness" and likely have as much joy and love as any other parent. However, there is one other significant difference. Parents of typical children look forward, with eagerness or trepidation, to the time when their child will no longer need their care, when the child takes responsibility for her own future. This may not be true for extreme caregivers.

Both Greenfeld and Brown, while they have adapted to the daily grind of caregiving, have also realized that the extent of the task is essentially unknowable. This suggests that, following the awful uncertainty of the child's heath in the early years, comes a phase where worries about the child's survival are replaced (or superseded) by worries about the child's future. In his later books, Greenfeld becomes much more pessimistic about Noah's future, as caring for him becomes steadily more difficult, and the horror and necessity of institutionalization looms (1978, 1986). For Brown, Walker's banishment to an institution is unthinkable, but so is continuing the enormous task of caring for him on a daily basis. It is difficult for him to think about the future, as it is clear that Walker's needs will not go away, and that Brown will not be able to fill them forever. However, these worries, like the earlier grief, are only an undercurrent of daily life. It is when a life-threatening illness or a new problem occurs that the future looms large. At that point, the conditions upon which the caregiving might stop are horrifying.

Some parents have been offered the option to escape from their caregiving burden by allowing an illness to take its natural course. When my brother was four years old, he caught pneumonia. My parents took him to the doctor, of course, and were told that they had two choices: to take him home or to put him in the hospital. On further questioning, it became obvious that hospitalization was the usual medical recommendation, and so that is what they chose. According to my father, the option to "take him home" was accompanied by a look of weighted sympathy, which he comprehended only much later as an unspoken opportunity to unburden himself by letting his son die of natural causes. While at times my father seemed to regret that he had not understood and taken the option, he also remained furious that he had been offered it.

Ian Brown had a similar experience. Early in *The Boy in the Moon*, when Walker is still an infant, fussy and not eating properly, but not yet diagnosed with CFC, his father takes him to see his pediatrician. Unknown to Brown, the pediatrician is aware that Walker has a major syndrome but has not yet identified it. He says to Brown, hinting that Walker's survival might require extraordinary means, "We do want this child to live, don't we?" Brown's answer, recounting the experience in the writing of the book, is:

> I decided it was a rhetorical question . . .. Even if he had asked it outright, I can't imagine my answer would have been anything but yes. All the ethical theorizing in the world can't change the pressures of the moment: the squalling baby on the examining table, his distended stomach, the doctor's obvious concern, his father standing gormlessly by. The call of the physical child and his need . . ..
>
> Criminal thoughts, or at least outlandish ones: what if we don't take extraordinary measures? What if he gets sick and we don't work so hard to get him better? Not murder, just nature. But even as I considered these grave plans, I knew I could never enact them. I'm not bragging; my hesitation wasn't ethical or moral. It was a more medieval urge, instinctual and physical; fear of a particular mode of failure, fear of retribution if I ignored the dull call of his flesh and his body and his need. (2011, p. 26).

Like my father, Brown was almost unable to recognize the doctor's suggestion. In fact, both of them might merely have imagined the incident. But later reflection relegates the asking of the question to a moral and guilt-ridden gray area. The decision that was never really made, or offered, still haunts him. Of course we want the child to live. When we have the resources and ability to save a life, why wouldn't we?

Brown likely speaks for many parents here. Despite his seeming uncertainty, his reaction is neither gormless nor hopeless. It springs from a sort of instinctual parental duty, which is a combination of an ancient response of a parent to a child's need and a modern expectation of how parents should behave. Though he might be tired and sometimes sad, he is mostly willing to take on the burden demanded of him, in part because the care of this particular child has fallen to him, but mostly because his love for that child is boundless.

I suspect that there are few, if any, parents who would agree to withholding treatment from a child in order to relieve their caregiving burden. For both Ian Brown and my father, the idea of enacting a plan that would lead to their child's death from medical causes was unthinkable, and the suggestion from professionals was met with resentment and horror. Both of them were working to live in peace with the burden they had shouldered, though we shall see in the next section that they were not always successful. Medical professionals did them a disservice when they imagined only the emotional burden and tried to craft for them a presumed escape from it.

With this in mind, the escape that we did not have a chance to offer Jeanette's father seems morally questionable. We thought of Jeanette's death as a relief from a terrible burden. For us, the worst had already happened, leaving behind a child whose life seemed to be comprised only of suffering. She certainly was suffering in the moment we saw her—she was critically ill, after all—yet, like my brother, her acute problem was a treatable pneumonia. Our reluctance to begin treatment was based on presumptions about her life outside the hospital; we could only imagine how difficult her care must be for her parents. We felt guilty for snatching her away from a death we felt appropriate and viewed with horror the continuation of a life we imagined as being terribly limited. But we had no idea how her father might feel about it. We did not know what her life meant to her family. I suspect that, to her father, Jeanette's death was unthinkable, perhaps a further unfairness to a child who had already been through too much. The emotional burden that her father was carrying, likely a combination of fear, guilt, and unconditional love, was entirely different from ours. He would not imagine her death as a welcome relief, even if he was, as we presumed, carrying an intolerable burden.

Living with Ambivalence: Dancing with Death

I have said that parents might resent offers from medical providers to allow a child to die, or might be angered at suggestions that death would be a welcome relief. But though parents say that they cannot bear the thought of a life without the child, they also often recognize for themselves that one of the ways out of this difficult duty is the death of the child. In order to introduce the ambivalence this can create, and how it affects the lives of extreme caregivers, I want to tell the story of a parent for whom death was always the only possible outcome.

Emily Rapp's son Ronan was diagnosed with Tay-Sachs disease at age nine months. She knew at once that this was a death sentence for him. He had already begun missing developmental milestones, and the presence of this disease meant that he would soon begin to regress. The course of Tay-Sachs disease is relentless and well-documented. Infants progressively lose neurological abilities until, eventually, their bodies can no longer function. Death usually occurs by age three, and there is no known cure.

Rapp decided to devote herself, for as long as necessary, to giving Ronan whatever life she could. Her memoir, *The Still Point of the Turning World* (2013), examines the meaning and experiences brought by Ronan's limited life. The ambiguity in this task is evident in its essential impossibility; she must give a life to a child who is dying, and create for him experiences that he will never be able to remember or understand. Rapp is quite frank about the ambiguity that caring for Ronan brought to her own life. She states, "In these moments, and when I lingered at the edge of the crib watching him breathe, I felt bottomless with sadness, each breath a fall into a trap door, and I also felt absolutely, euphorically alive" (p. 184).

She also admits to an even larger ambiguity about Ronan's life; she'd had prenatal screening for Tay-Sachs, which had failed to detect his particular genetic defect. She knows that she would have had an abortion to prevent his birth if the test had been accurate and she'd been aware of the diagnosis. Challenged about this, in an interview on National Public Radio, just after the book's publication (and Ronan's death), Rapp stated that the life Ronan had was not something she would have chosen for him, or for herself. She could, however, be grateful that Ronan was her child and, at the same time, wish that he'd never been born. This was, she asserted, "a duality that could be held" (Rapp, NPR, 2013).

Several of the papers on caring for medically complex children at home contain brief summaries of the ambivalent emotions that parents sometimes reported. Nursing scholar Berit Brinchmann, after conducting interviews with several families living with a severely disabled child, concluded that ambivalence in the parents' relationships to their children was a major theme. She stated, "The children are utterly dependent upon their parents, who both love and hate their children . . .. The parents lack relief from the situation . . .. This and their total dependence create strong bonds between them, including an experience of love and adoration. Every day is full of contrasts, full of both sorrow and sadness, but also of love and happiness" (1999, p. 141). These parents, like Emily Rapp, seemed to be holding the duality of living with two conflicting emotions at the same time.

Some of the parents seemed to regret the child's birth, stating that "they would have had an abortion or terminated the treatment for their child if they had known how serious the handicap was going to be," but those same parents also "expressed that their lives with these children had given them something positive, something precious, which they would not have experienced otherwise" (Brinchmann, 1999, p. 141). These parents, too, could be grateful for their child's existence while still regretting the child's birth.

Their regret was partly motivated by recognizing the suffering their child had to endure because of her disabilities. But parents also regretted the enormous burden of care that they faced. Though they felt trapped by that burden, and sometimes wished they were out of the trap, they recognized that the burden came with a child that they loved. Another parent said that "losing her [child] would be so much more emotionally painful than the burden of having her" (Brinchmann, 1999, p. 141). The bonds formed between parent and extremely dependent child were not negated by the realization that life for their child, and for themselves, was difficult.

Families of children on home ventilators experience similarly complicated emotional reactions to their children's extreme need. They must balance a complex tension between positive and negative emotions, which one researcher called "daily living with distress and enrichment." The worry, fear, isolation, and burden of work are balanced by "deep enrichments and rewarding experiences that they could not imagine living without" (Carnevale, et al., 2006, p. e53) These parents at times wondered if keeping their child alive by starting home ventilation had been the right decision yet also stated that life without the child would be unthinkable. They might regret the life they find themselves living, but that life does hold rewarding moments and love for the child.

During times of despair, some parents feel that there is seemingly no end to the burdens they have taken on. In the absence of adequate respite care and with a dire shortage of long-term care facilities, parents cannot look forward to relief from their caregiving burdens. Nor do they have an answer for the awful question of who will care for their child when they cannot possibly continue doing it. The parents of a child who might never become independent, will realize that the only way out of this uncertain future is death, either the child's or their own. Both are unthinkable. But sometimes that despair, grounded in love for the child, takes the form of a desire to protect the child from this seemingly bleak future.

My father had a fantasy, that he confessed to me on several occasions over about twenty years, of a way to solve the problem of my brother's long-term care. He and my mother were finding it increasingly difficult to care for Paul, and they did not want to have to burden anyone else with it. His fantasy was that he would go for a drive with Paul and, at a place where it was likely to be fatal, just drive off the road. They both would be killed in the fiery wreck. Problem solved! He was quite serious, and I was never entirely sure he wouldn't do it. But of course he never did. He loved his son, was proud of the things that Paul learned to do against all odds, and would not have encouraged his death.

As he confesses in his book *Without Reason*, Charles Hart had a similar plan when he first learned that his child Ted was "brain damaged." (The diagnosis of autism did not become clear until years later.) Hart knew of the life of "humiliation, grief, and frustration" that his son could expect, because of his experiences with his own brother, Sumner, who likewise suffered from this yet unidentified problem. "Our beautiful child had ceased to be a source of hope and pride," he recalls, "Instead he had become a source of pain, a burden that would grow greater with time. I immediately foresaw the worst, Ted growing unmanageable and unkempt, disfigured and rejected by society" (1989, p. 44). Hart, like my father, had a solution. "A plan formed in my mind. We could take a ride on one of our state ferries. When the ship cruised into the deep waters of Puget Sound I would hold my son close to me and jump overboard. Our suffering wouldn't last long . . ." (p. 46). Yet Hart's love for his son is undeniably present throughout his book.

Josh Greenfeld, does not express a murder/suicide fantasy in *A Child Called Noah*, but he does admit to thinking, "There's simply no way out. I must confess something: sometimes I hope Noah gets sick and dies painlessly" (1970, p. 139). However, Noah's brother Karl has recently written his own memoir about growing up with Noah. In *Boy Alone*, Karl Taro Greenfeld reports that his father, in both conversations and interviews, did talk about killing Noah (2009). According to Karl, Josh Greenfeld's scenarios mostly involved allowing Noah to fall overboard from a boat. All he would have had to do was take Noah for a boat ride and forget to put him in a life vest.

Later, as Noah became older and more difficult to control, Josh Greenfeld publicly advocated euthanasia for people with severe autism. But, Karl stresses, "my mother and father love Noah as any parents love their son" (K. Greenfeld, 2009, p. 219). It is likely that Josh Greenfeld saw the same bleak future that Hart imagined for his son: a life of unhappiness, poor care, and rejection. As Noah grew without improvement, Greenfeld felt that Noah's death might be preferable to the horrors of institutional care that were closing in on him. He seemed torn between terrible alternatives, but he did not really want to become a murderer in order to spare his son from a fate worse than death. Karl explains, "My father used to tell me that he talked and wrote about killing Noah because that meant he could never do it, that the confession and motive were already there, on tape, in his books, so he could never get away with the crime" (K. Greenfeld, 2009, p. 338).

Hart and Greenfeld both had experiences with the institutional system. Hart's older brother Sumner was moved between several care facilities when his mother could no longer care for him in the 1970s. The abuses and misunderstandings he suffered fill several chapters and include refusing to eat, losing the ability to care for himself, smearing himself with feces, and running away. Noah Greenfeld's experiences with day and residential care in a variety of settings began in the same decade. Noah also experienced deprivation and corporal punishment (in the name of operant conditioning), and he expressed his unhappiness and outrage with violent behavior. I believe that, rather than blaming the fathers for their dark thoughts, we must instead continue to work to ensure that the future for Noah, Sumner, and others like them, does not become as bleak as their fathers imagined it might be.

Ian Brown (2011) is even more inventive than either Hart or Greenfeld, and his scenarios are even darker. He dedicates several pages to fantasies about a way out for Walker and himself. He has not seen any possibility of passing Walker's care to someone else, and it is clear that his main intent is to end his own exhausting and seemingly endless caregiving burden.

> On especially difficult nights, or if it rained hard, or most of all after the terrible arguments my wife and I sometimes had, strained by sleeplessness and ashamed of our failure with this strange boy, I asked myself if it might not be braver to take my life, and to take Walker with me. Suicide is not my default setting. But the hopelessness of life ahead, caring for Walker, could raise the spectre in me. There was chloral hydrate; there were pills. There was the car, there were places to drive the car off of, there were lakes to walk into. (p. 223)

Another plan is worrisome in its precision and detail:

> One of my secret death fantasies was to pack Walker into a baby backpack I owned, a kind of Snugli, and take him high up into the mountains of western Canada in the winter, one of my favourite places on earth, and lie down in a snowbank, and end it there, quietly, hypothermically.

> I imagined the venture in complete detail, how I would pick a moment when Johanna [his wife] was at a movie and Hayley [his daughter] was at school, how I would get him out of the house and to the airport, with all his gear and all the ski equipment. Unfortunately that alone derailed my death fantasy: if I could get through that fucking nightmare, the airport with Walker and skis, I could survive anything, and there was no need to kill myself. (p. 224)

Of course, Brown does not carry out any of it. I think it is interesting that even his fantasy suicide pact falls apart because he is just too tired from the daily round of caregiving. He can imagine every detail of the plan, including exactly how difficult and frustrating it would be to carry it out. Not only that, but if it is possible to travel with all that gear while also caring for Walker, it is also possible to carry out the daily grind at home for another day. Instead of killing himself and Walker, he resigns himself, not just to keep going but also to keep trying to make a future for Walker and a life for himself outside of Walker's needs.

Yet he finds joy in Walker also. On one of those dark nights, exhausted, he falls down the steps while carrying Walker. Walker thinks it's hilarious. "He laughed. Loved it. And so, I did too. He took me into darkness but he was often the way out of it as well" (p. 226.) His love for Walker is palpable, and wrenching. Early in the book, just after the nightmarish night wakening, Walker falls asleep in Brown's arms. Brown writes, "I long for the moment when he lets his crazy, formless body fall asleep against me . . . . Sometimes I think this is his gift to me—parceled out, to show me how rare and valuable it is. Walker, my teacher, my sweet, sweet, lost and broken boy" (p. 7).

Clearly the narratives of death or murder or suicide are not evidence of lack of love toward the child. But what meaning might they express? Anthropologist Cheryl Mattingly, in an ethnographic study of mothers of critically ill children, has proposed that the presence of a severe, potentially fatal illness places mothers in a position in which they must live with several, conflicting (or downright mutually exclusive) life narratives. She believes that sorting through these possibilities is a necessary moral undertaking. Mothers of children with life-threatening illnesses must begin to process the child's death, while simultaneously living day-to-day in hope that the child will recover and live. One mother in the study erected a very strong narrative of hope from both medical information and religious beliefs, which helped her to support herself and her child. Yet she also befriended a mother whose child was actively dying of the same illness.

Mattingly says that this mother's "insistence" on hope was "belied by her simultaneous efforts to face an opposing future story, creating experiences and taking actions that compel her to recognize a much darker possibility" (2014, p. 133). This moral action allowed her later to face her own daughter's death from a position of strength.

I believe that it is the need to recognize a "much darker possibility" that motivates the imaginations of Brown, Greenfeld, Hart, and my father. They are fortifying themselves, not against death, but against a future in which their child is not loved or even cared for. There must be some comfort in imagining an ending where the future is known, and their child will not have to live through rejection or neglect, though death is indeed a drastic way to solve the problem. Yet none of them, with the exception of Greenfeld, can imagine such a solution in the absence of their own deaths as well.

Rapp lived a somewhat different set of competing narratives. She never, from the moment of diagnosis, imagined any outcome other than death for her son Ronan. Knowing that Ronan's neurologic disease would take him from being unable to develop, through being unable to respond, to being, in the end, barely conscious, she set out to narrate for him a full and meaningful, though short, life. She did not oppose narratives between life and death but sought a new definition of life.

Rapp recalls,

> As tragic as the situation appeared from the outside, the inside of our lives was often blissful, despite the daily very real dread about what was happening as this ridiculous disease spread across Ronan's brain and shut down his body. In the morning we lifted Ronan from his crib and kissed him. There was joy. We laughed. We lived. I took him hiking and rubbed his fat feet in the dirt and lifted his face to the juniper-scented breeze. He went on road trips, to parties, coffee shops and restaurants. He was our companion, our child, our beloved. (2013, pp. 24–25)

And yet, he was dying, not in some decade so far in the future as to be irrelevant, but right then, by sometimes detectable degrees, as his nerves shut down, taking him further away every day.

In encounters with clinicians, parents often seem to be either struggling and falling into despair, or eagerly monitoring and championing their child's progress. I suspect that parents actually live day-to-day with both realities, and that they show clinicians whichever one the parent thinks the clinician wishes to see. They must walk a line between failing to cope and being in denial. We saw in the previous chapter that parents were suspected of emphasizing the positive when participating in quality of life studies, because that is what they thought the researchers wanted to hear, and also that parents seemingly emphasize the positive in parent support groups and online chat rooms (Harrison, 2001). I suspect that parents who want urgent respite care or additional services must do the opposite, and express their desperation as failure to cope. None of these parents are lying, merely emphasizing different truths. It is both unnecessary and unfair to ask them to consistently demonstrate one truth all of the time.

Extreme caregiving parents must maintain a foothold in competing truths. They must live daily with both distress and enrichment. They must, often at the same time, wish that things had been different and embrace the way things are. They must balance despair and hope, grief and joy. They can, as Emily Rapp did, simultaneously wish that the child had not been born and cherish every moment with him. They can, as Ian Brown did, wish for the terrible burden of care to end and fervently hope their child will never know pain or rejection. The child and the burden of caring for the child are inseparable. It is a duality which can be held. Indeed, it is a duality which must be held. It may be that upholding it is one of the most difficult moral tasks undertaken in extreme caregiving.

Advocacy and the Maintenance of Value

I have said that parents sometimes deal with the emotional journey on which they have embarked by imagining the darker possibilities in their child's future. It is far more common, however, for parents to promote a positive narrative, as they imagine, and work to bring into reality, the best possible future for their child. Creating the best possible future often requires both personal growth and public advocacy, in order to recognize and promote the value of a child whose disabilities may diminish him in the eyes of the world. It is so necessary that I am including it as one of the unrecognized responsibilities of raising a child with special needs.

The responsibilities I will be addressing here concern the day-to-day navigation of a new reality, one that contains a child who is not what was expected, by either the parent or the rest of the world. It is a process that requires both creativity and imagination, as a parent constructs a new life, a new "normal," out of the necessity to expand their old expectations and encompass the life of a child with extra needs. The parents must first change themselves and then, often, bring the rest of the world into line.

In the Preface, I spoke about Emily Perl Kingsley's essay "Welcome to Holland," a metaphor for living with a child with disabilities. I believe Kingsley is correct in emphasizing that parents have arrived in a new and different world, and that this new world can hold unexpected happiness. I disagree with the implication that this new world is easy to recognize and relatively easy to navigate. Extreme caregivers must create, perhaps out of the ashes of dashed expectations, a new world in which to live. Their discovery begins with the child and the care that child requires, and includes the process of learning to accept and value the child. Ultimately they must build a home and a world where the child and the family can thrive.

Beginning at the moment when parents first suspect that something is wrong—often before they receive a diagnosis or know what that diagnosis means for the future of their family—parents must learn to cope with new information and expectations. They must work to create themselves as new people who can do what must be done to raise a child with special needs. They must not only work to learn the new tasks of care, from changing diapers to using medical technology, but also learn to navigate the confusing and conflicting feelings that inevitably arise. As they find a path through the emotional ups and downs of diagnosis, and the acceptance of medical realities, they must readjust their expectations for developmental progress and success. As they care for the child at home, they must create a safe haven where the child's limitations are normal and accepted. An enormous part of this task hinges on accepting and valuing the child for who she is, disabilities notwithstanding.

As part of forging their new lives, parents must often work in opposition to a social narrative of disability as unwanted and unlivable, and people with disabilities as without value. They also must reinvent themselves as caregivers in a society where caregiving is both invisible and devalued. In overcoming their own preconceived ideas about disability, parents often also find themselves on the front lines of a social battle for acceptance and respect for their child.

One common social narrative that parents, particularly mothers, must work against, is the expectation of perfection. A recent *Time* magazine poll reports, "nearly 80% of millennial moms [defined as born in the late 70's to early 90's] say it's important to be 'the perfect mom'," a much higher proportion than the previous two generations of mothers (Steinmetz, 2015). Being the perfect mother implies monitoring bodily health during pregnancy, following all medical advice, and acting as a model parent once the child is born. It also means that the child, a reflection on her mother, must meet certain standards of perfection.

At a time when it seems possible to avoid having a baby with certain genetic characteristics, and when it is seen as desirable to someday be able to design a baby to improved specifications, mothers seem to be expected to produce the best children possible. The public narrative surrounding reproduction suggests that control of the outcome of pregnancy is already scientifically possible, if the mother complies with all current recommendations. Mothers who produce a child who does not meet expectations are suspected by society of having done something wrong, either by failing to follow all medical advice during pregnancy or by refusing genetic testing. The mother is thus given the responsibility for producing the best possible baby, by exercising "her obligation to undergo prenatal screening and selective abortion of defective fetuses and through her control of the uterine environment" (Landsman, 1998, p. 80).

In the eyes of many in this medicalized world, having a child with a potentially detectable genetic syndrome is seen as either an accident that could have easily been avoided or a selfish, impractical choice. Mothers of children with Down syndrome report being questioned, by both medical staff and casual acquaintances, about the reasons they neglected to have prenatal testing or chose not to abort an effected fetus (Lalvani, 2011). This is true for mothers of children with other genetic diseases as well. Emily Rapp, whose son had a rare form of Tay-Sachs disease that is not routinely included in screening, also reports being challenged on her presumed failure to have the proper testing done (Rapp, 2013). And so, even before the life of the child with disabilities begins, that child's life has been judged by society—and found wanting.

Essentially, this attitude forces a mother who has a child with disabilities to feel that she has already failed in motherhood by producing an imperfect child. Gail Landsman (1999), anthropologist and mother of a daughter with disabilities, interviewed twenty-one mothers of children with disabilities, and found that mothers not only felt blame from others, but blamed themselves, often reviewing their own actions or examining themselves for suspect activities that might have led to the disability. They expressed "a sense of profound injustice and betrayal" (1999, p. 142) at having a disabled child though they had done nothing wrong. Mothers of children with many forms of disability have to work away from this narrative in which a less than perfect baby makes them into an inadequate mother. To resist the blame that has been assigned to them, they must reconstruct what it means to be a mother, discovering in themselves deeper skills and commitments.

One narrative that resists blame is to ascribe to the mother special abilities or powers, which explain why she was "chosen" for a task that, perhaps, no one else would be able to accomplish. Landsman also asked the mothers about the common sentiment that "God gives special kids to special parents." Some mothers were able to silence doubts by thinking that they had been singled out as special. In the narrative of specialness, Landsman says, "The mother shifts from being defined as a careless producer of a defective product to a purposely chosen recipient of a special gift" (1999, p. 142).

At later interviews, however, many of the mothers were beginning to reject that narrative, for various reasons. Some understood that while having a disabled child did eventually make them different from other people, they did not start out any better or worse than other parents. They were not saints and were not singled out because they were either particularly special or the reverse, in need of special instruction. Some mothers rejected the narrative of specialness because it glosses over the difficulties of raising a child with special needs. One mother, talking about this sort of "platitude," states, "It just diminishes . . . the adversity. It belittles it. It undermines what you've been through" (Landsman, 1999, p. 145).

Landsman also rejects the specialness narrative because it, "maintains intact the belief in the possibility of quality control, [and] also supports both the cultural mandate to have perfect babies and the 'othering' of disabled children and the mothers who give birth to them" (1999, p. 142). Mothers in another study agreed. They rejected the message of their own specialness because saying that their child required a sort of super-parent could be perceived as diminishing the value of the child (Lalvani, 2011). I agree that attributing special abilities to the mother contributes to the social narrative of perfection and devalues the child and the mother. It also diminishes any difficult caregiving work the mother is doing.

Implicit in the narratives of both tragedy and blame is an idea that the child with disabilities is less desirable than other children because of the disability (Lalvani, 2011). The disabled, or "defective," child is seen as being not only a burden to the parents but also inherently of lesser value than a typical child. Another way that parents resist this is to ascribe special abilities or value, not to themselves, but to the child. Usually this is done by reframing the child as an exceptional person who has not only exceeded the dim expectations of worthlessness provided by doctors or society but also has bestowed priceless gifts upon anyone who truly comes to know the child. By "redefining her child neither as a product nor as a gift from God, but as a *giver* of gifts, a mother of a child with disabilities raises the value of her child beyond that of the 'perfect' child she had once expected to acquire" (Landsman, 1999, 148).

This narrative is repeated multiple times in the book *Gifts: Mothers Reflect on How Children with Down Syndrome Enrich Their Lives*, a collection of essays by sixty-three mothers of children with Down syndrome (Soper, 2007). The stated intent of the collection is to provide reassurance to mothers who have recently been informed that their child has Down syndrome. Not surprisingly, the story the essays tell is similar. Most mothers begin by describing their attitude prior to receiving the diagnosis. Some are sure they would never be able to parent such a child, or convinced that such parenting would be awful, or secretly believe that children with disabilities are of lesser value than typical children. When they find out they indeed have a child with Down syndrome, they are devastated. But then they come to realize the enormous gifts their child has brought them. Those gifts are, in chapter order: respect, strength, delight, perspective, and love. They find in themselves the ability to see value in everyone and the strength to fight for their child's needs. They find personal growth in reorienting their priorities, and they delight in the love they have for their children (and their children for them).

Michael Berube, a professor of literature, disability activist, and father of a twenty-six-year-old son with Down syndrome, resists this common narrative. He introduces his new book about his son, *Life as Jamie Knows It*, with this statement,

> [W]e will not tell you that Jamie is a sweet angel/cherub whose plucky triumphs over disability inspire us all. We will not tell you that special-needs children are gifts sent to special parents. And we will definitely not tell you that God never gives someone more than he or she can handle, because, as a matter of fact, God does that all the time. (Berube, 2016, p 16)

Neither Jamie nor his parents are particularly special. However, like other parents, Berube finds life with his son "far richer than we could have imagined before Jamie was born" (p 16). While parents do find in themselves new strengths, reordered priorities, and intense love for their child, those things come, not from the child, but from the daily necessity to make a life for the child.

I am suspicious of the use of the narrative of gifts to establish social value for any child with disabilities. In much the same way that the narrative of parental specialness supports the cultural mandate to produce perfect babies, the narrative of the child as the bearer of special gifts upholds the cultural message that worth is established by ability and action. Asking parents to reinforce this narrative is essentially asking the parent to figure out for us a value for their child. Their children are valued only if they can be seen to supply a special service. Fighting for the value of life with disabilities by finding special abilities that only the disabled might provide, seems to me to be self-defeating. Perhaps it would be more useful to fight for a reorientation of what is considered valuable.

The advocacy that these parents are called upon to do includes working to establish a better definition of social value. It is well worth paying attention to the new, improved definition that has come from their experiences and intimate knowledge. Does God give special kids to special parents? No, but the journey into this strange world does result in a different viewpoint. Parents were not selected for their specialness, but they do become special, or at least different, with new sensibilities and values. Extreme caregiving does not require you to be a special person in advance, but it does make you into one.

If children are measured by the usual methods—academic and financial success, perhaps—those with disabilities, particularly intellectual disabilities, will seem inadequate. But their parents do not view them as having lesser value. And so they learn to celebrate success in new places, and find joy in, perhaps, first steps at age seven or toilet training at age eleven. Many say that they have become better, happier people by giving up their earlier expectations and adapting to the slower pace of their child's development. Instead of looking toward grades and the preparation for a high-earning job, parents focus on the capacity, in themselves and in the child, to learn acceptance, respect, joy, and love. In learning to accept their child, "not in spite of or because of the disability but simply with it as an integral part of who he/she is" (Green, 2007, p. 157), they learn a different set of priorities and acquire a deeper understanding of value. We will return in Chapter 7 to the new values learned through extreme caregiving.

They also learn that they must spread their understanding to teach others to value their child as they do. Many parents join in the battle for diversity, social change, and acceptance of people with disabilities, though it is not a mandatory part of extreme caregiving.

The need for advocacy on a personal level is almost unavoidable, however. It is a responsibility one receives along with caring for the child. Another mother of a child with Down syndrome likens the new world she entered with her son's birth to a college degree program. Advocacy is an advanced class. She writes,

> Advocacy 203: When I first saw the title of this class I assumed it would require rousing speeches, fist pounding, and the making of demands on my son's behalf. It all seemed very intimidating. What I learned, however, was that advocacy could mean something as small as taking my son to the mall and letting him be a baby as unremarkable as any of the other babies in their strollers on a quiet weekday morning. (Bremer, 2007, pp. 88–89)

Political action, strident or otherwise, is not the only form advocacy takes. Sometimes advocacy is necessary when the disapproval of strangers turns an ordinary encounter at the mall into a moral crisis. Parents must sometimes try to try bridge the gulf that has distanced them from others, and teach others to see the child through their eyes. They must also learn when it is better to walk away. Clashes, sometimes heartbreaking, occur regularly. Sometimes it is necessary to change the world by one single, gentle encounter at a time.

The need for advocacy in both medicine and politics is fairly obvious. It is necessary in schools and communities when appropriate services are not available. It comes in encounters with the medical system when uninsured treatments must be fought for, or professionals under- (or over-) estimate their child's potential. But it is in the personal realm where the most difficult work must be done. While creating a home and a world where their child's needs are met, parents must remake themselves as well. Like the parents who wrote about coming to terms with Down syndrome, perhaps they must learn to see value in diversity or redefine their ideas of success. Certainly they must reset their priorities as they adjust to a life that revolves around meeting the multiple and complex needs of their child. We would do well to learn these things from them. We should help them wherever possible to create a society where care is noticed and valued, and where success is measured by acceptance rather than by the amount of revenue a person can generate.

Lack of Choice

A great deal of attention is given, these days, particularly in the medical ethics (or bioethics) literature, to the matter of personal choice. Through the first principle of bioethics, autonomy, we are all to understand that we can exert control over what happens to us. However, in many circumstances, that control is mere illusion. Very few people set out in pregnancy with the goal of having a child with disabilities. A few are offered, through prenatal screening, the decision to end a pregnancy, "preventing" the birth of a child with a genetic syndrome. We have seen that the possibility of this decision, and the illusion of control it offers, has societal consequences with repercussions felt by all parents of children with disabilities. But, of course, parents do not often choose the child who is born nor how many problems he or she might have. They also do not have much choice when it comes time to care for the child's special needs at home.

The choices available to these parents, while perhaps couched in the trappings of autonomous choice, are not truly viable choices. As for the question posed earlier, "We do want this child to live, don't we?" there is really only one answer: Yes. The follow-up question, the one that makes parents into extreme caregivers, is, "We do want to this child to go home, don't we?" Home is where children are supposed to be, where they thrive and grow up. Of course we want the child to go home.

In part, we want the child to go home because we have created no alternatives, no other places where the child might thrive. When my brother was diagnosed with what was at that time referred to as mental retardation, my parents were offered, and expected to take, the option of placing him in an institution. At the time, many felt this to be a reasonable choice, perhaps because they were unaware of the inadequacy of care in the institutions. Those who were aware seemed to think that raising such a child was either impossible or so difficult that it was not worth doing. Some upscale institutions for children of the wealthy existed, but for many with fewer financial resources, institutionalization really meant a slow decline from neglect. This was the case at our local institution, Pennhurst, and sending my brother there was not a reasonable choice for my parents. There was no other option available.

Those horrible institutions have since been shut down, but there are still few options other than caring for the child at home. Children with complex needs can be placed in a nursing home or hospital, but neither is ideal. Adequate nursing home care for a child is hard to find and can be prohibitively expensive. Having a child in a hospital or care facility for an extended period also divides the family between two different and sometimes distant locations. I have seen children live in the hospital for prolonged periods, usually because they are too unstable to go home. As the months stretch by, it becomes more difficult for parents to continue daily involvement, and the family drifts apart. A few children are placed in medical foster care, but most parents consider this a punishment for inadequacy, and few parents want this to happen (Mattingly, 2014).

Some parents of ventilator-dependent children have been given the choice to take a child home on a ventilator or remove airway support and let the child die. In a 2011 study of the ethical challenges of home mechanical ventilation (HMV), some of the parents reported that they "asked themselves whether they made the right decision, but in reality, they did not have other choices if the alternative was to let their child die" (Dwybik, 2011, p. 240). Most of the children in this study had a progressive neurological disease, and perhaps were being offered HMV as a life-extending therapy in the face of death. Some feel that prolonging life in this manner is so uncomfortable for the child that death is preferable; many parents do not agree. In this circumstance, a hospital might recommend transfer, but many communities do not have facilities that can care for a child on a ventilator. It is likely that a lack of alternatives to home care contributed to a parental understanding that their only option was to choose to care for the child on a ventilator at home.

I believe that cost is also driving care toward the home. There is a widespread perception that home care is cheaper. But, as we have seen, some researchers believe that home care seems cheaper only because the extraneous costs, borne by the family, are not taken into account (Kirk, 1998). We have seen that parents provide a great deal of unpaid labor, at a high financial cost to themselves in lost wages. Researchers who performed a cost analysis of family caregiving for children with special health care needs (CSHCN) concluded that "family provided health care represents a critical component of the health care system for CSHCN," and that if parents "were to stop or significantly reduce the amount of care they provided, major gaps in health care would be exposed" (Romley et al., 2017). I doubt that children are being inappropriately forced out of the hospital and into the home, but parents pay the invisible, or unaccounted for, costs of care when they agree to care for a child at home.

However, most parents make the decision to assume care at home because, in medical estimation and in their own, regardless of cost, home is understood to be the best place for a child to be. Discharge to home has become part of the presumed medical best interest of the disabled and chronically ill child. The parent is expected to provide whatever care is necessary. Though it is offered to parents as a decision they must make, the parent is charged with making a decision that promotes the best interests of the child. If home is indeed the best place for the child to be, the choice to become an extreme caregiver is then merely a matter of deciding when and how home care will be accomplished.

In a pediatric paper exploring ethical issues around home care, pediatric ethicist John Lantos asserts that it is paramount that any decision to discharge a child to home care be clearly in the child's best interest. His ethical qualms center on establishing the home as the best place for the child, a place where she will get the best care at the lowest cost. He acknowledges the difficulty this might pose for the parents. He states, "On the one hand, if home care is both cheaper and more beneficial for the child than long-term hospital or institutional care, it would seem to be ethically imperative. However, the benefits of home care are uniquely sensitive to the voluntariness of parental participation" (1992, p. 922). Lantos maintains that in order to meet ethical guidelines, the families must understand what they are getting into, meet established competence standards, and agree on the goals of home care. However, while Lantos does state that the child's needs must be balanced against the family's needs, and that parents should not be judged unacceptable if they are unable or unwilling to carry out home care, he does not explore the nature of the "voluntariness" of the parental decision.

At this time, parents are expected to voluntarily take on home care as part of promoting the best interest of the child. Some ethicists are bothered by this paradox, and feel that the interests of the child (or the patient) should not always be paramount. Speaking about both pediatric and adult patients requiring home technology, John Arras, a philosopher and professor of bioethics, argues that the interests of other family members should also be taken into account. He says, "the systematic exclusion of the interests of family and friends who provide care at home is untenable and unjust" (1994, p. s24). He feels that parents, when asked to provide home care, are not really allowed to refuse, lest they be seen as uncaring or bad parents. Parents also see that there are no viable alternatives to home care and few options for long-term hospitalization or long-term care facilities. Arras states, "Unless families have access to such alternatives, their initial acceptance of the home care plan becomes a trap from which there is no practical escape" (1994, p. s25).

But most parents of children who require prolonged hospitalization for any reason, long for the day when the child will be discharged. In part, they look forward to a homecoming when their lives will return to normal—as though coming home and being cured are the same. Many of the narratives of premature birth actually end with that happy homecoming, and play down or ignore the possibility of continuing medical problems (Smith, 1999; Woodwell, 2001; Fei, 2015). But even when a child is obviously not cured at the time of discharge, parents still desperately want the child at home. They know that it is the best place the child can be, where he will be loved and appreciated and cared for. But though they eagerly and voluntarily take on that caregiving, they cannot know what they are getting into.

Once the child is at home, and the true nature and amount of care required is finally realized, the parents do not have an opportunity to reverse their decision. With the absence of alternative placement and respite care, parents are on their own. Many of the parents in Lynne Ray's study of the parents of chronically ill children reported that their only choice was between "falling apart" or "getting on with the show" (Ray, 2002, p. 433). They just kept going, because there was no alternative. Parents in Berit Brinchmann's study of severely impaired NICU survivors living at home came to a similar conclusion. Several parents reported that they now regretted their decision, but as Brinchmann puts it, "One cannot decide against something one already has" (1999, p. 141).

A mother of a child with Down syndrome summed up the problem: "You have no choice. This is it. You know, either you give them up, send them away to a home or you deal with it. It's not in between. I choose to deal with it" (Landsman, 1999, p. 144). Another mother, caring for a son with a neurodegenerative disease, stated of her choice to care for him at home, "He needs you. You are his mother. This is your task, hellish as it might be. You have no choice" (Rapp, 2013, p. 48).

Ian Brown takes on the involuntary nature of his caregiving duties with ironic resignation. After his son survives an early illness, he writes, "I felt like an ox slipping into its yoke. I could feel the heavy tragic years coming on ahead of me, as certain as bad weather" (2011, p. 27). Josh Greenfeld, on several occasions, usually associated with events that had been particularly trying, wished to end his caregiving duties. After a day of regression in toilet training, he remembers thinking about placing Noah in an institution. He writes, "Perhaps we ought to get rid of Noah. No, that would not solve anything. There are always demanding madnesses in one's life. No, that's a madness too: to make of Noah a metaphor. But as Noah gets old . . ." (1970, p. 107). He understands that institutionalization would put Noah into a precarious care situation, out of his sight but not out of his concern. He does not consider institutionalization a reasonable choice and so sees no way out of his current predicament. Both fathers also allude to the future, when caregiving will become ever more difficult, as both father and son get older. We return to this topic at length in Chapter 8.

Perhaps because preserving the best interests of the child is considered to be one of the many responsibilities assumed by parents, few ethical accounts include the moral work a parent must do to put their own interests aside and do what is best for the child. Cheryl Mattingly believes that the moral journey taken by the parent of a sick child is far more perilous and complex than we might expect. She reports on the dilemma of a mother of a child who requires multiple surgeries following severe accidental burns. The mother has to provide consent for the procedures, a medically trivial event. However, Mattingly says,

> [The mother] presents the problem of making the right decision not as a matter of willing something, of making a choice at a particular moment, as much as taking on the larger task of how to be the kind of person capable of facing such tough choices, acting from a position where she has the moral strength to perceive and act on the best good. It is the cultivation of a particular way of being a mother for her son that she sees as her bigger task. (2014, pp. 85–86)

To become a new kind of person capable of making the right decision is not a trivial journey. The choices offered are not truly choices at all, forcing her to become a different person in order to make them. Other parents also must learn to be a different kind of person, one who can deal with the child's problems and do what is best for the child. They must develop the moral strength to choose to keep their child's needs at the center of their lives.

Taking on the possibly endless burden of extreme caregiving is not really a choice when love or duty permits no other course of action. These parents are in many ways being forced into caregiving, which they neither expected nor chose to do. But the existence of the child is undeniable, and the vulnerability of his needs seems to supersede the desires of the parent. In some ways, the parents truly are, as the parent narrators often express, condemned as guilty for the child's problems. Unwillingly, or not, the parents become the people they have to be in order to carry out their new responsibilities.

If, as Tronto (1993) has proposed, attentiveness and taking responsibility are virtues that define the first two phases of caring, parents have a difficult moral journey ahead. To become attentive and responsible, they must balance an extraordinary number of needs. They must spend their lives monitoring their children's needs, and become attentive to too many things. Perhaps they have been given responsibility for far more than they can accomplish. Perhaps their own lives and concerns have been subsumed in the needs of their children, and they have put aside too many of their own needs and desires. They cannot avoid overindulgence and overcommitment while performing a task that might consume all of their time.

As the science of medicine has progressed, the number and complexity of parental responsibilities has grown, but, since parents have always been the default caregivers, there has been no reassessment of their duties. Within Tronto's (1993) phases of care, there is no necessity for all of the phases to be carried out by a single individual caregiver, be it nurse or physician or parent. There is no reason to make the parents of special needs children compromise themselves in order to carry out every part of the task of caring for their children. Overcommitment cannot be a failure on the parent caregiver's part; it is a societal failure of attentiveness. Likewise, those parents who seem not to be coping well are not failing in their responsibility. Instead, we as a medical system and a society have not taken on the responsibilities that we have helped create. We are not paying sufficient attention to the needs of either the child or the caregiver, nor taking sufficient responsibility for the care of the children whose existence is made possible by modern medicine.

Becoming the kind of person they need to be in order to care for their child—beginning by developing the virtues of attentiveness and responsibility—is difficult moral work. Parents must learn to live with the uncertainty of grief and guilt, while still hoping for the best for their child. They must live with the ambiguity of the loss of the child they expected and the gain of the child they have and cherish. They must recognize the value in their children and often defend that value in the face of a disapproving world. And they must learn to value themselves in their new role as extreme caregiver. Then, to make a place for the child to grow and thrive in the world, they must teach others what they have learned.

In the next phase of care, caregiving, we will consider parental competence in the act of meeting the needs for which extreme caregiving parents become responsible. For the child to thrive, the hands-on tasks of caregiving must be done, and must be done well. To meet their responsibilities, parents must acquire a wide range of competencies despite a great deal of variability in their education and natural abilities. We shall also see that both parents and professionals overlook this competence, as the day-to-day tasks of caregiving become secondary to the overarching need to help the child reach her highest potential.

CHAPTER 6 | Competence

IN THE PREVIOUS chapter, I reviewed how parenting a child who requires extreme caregiving differs from typical parenting, considering mostly the first two phases of care: "caring about" and "taking care of." We expect all parents to demonstrate the virtues associated with these two phases—attentiveness and responsibility. However, the heightened level of attentiveness and larger number of responsibilities we place on the parents of a child with special needs increases the emotional and moral work they must perform. In this chapter we consider the third phase of care, caregiving. This is the phase in which the actual hands-on work of meeting needs is done. The virtue associated with the third phase is competence, the ability to do the work which must be done, and to do it well. Given the number of new tasks which must be taken on, it will come as no surprise that parents in this phase must rise to a high level of competence.

Within Tronto's theory of care, competence becomes a moral action that can be evaluated by its effectiveness at meeting needs. If the actions of caregiving are done incompetently, the care provided is inadequate. "Intending to provide care, even accepting responsibility for it, but then failing to provide good care, means that in the end the need for care is not met" (Tronto, 1993, p. 133). Caregiving is the heart of care, the phase in which the actions necessary to provide for a need are taken. These actions must be done competently or care has not been accomplished.

All parents are expected to care for their children competently, but we have few guidelines to evaluate their effectiveness. There is, of course, no particular training for the task, nor is any organization assigned the responsibility for overseeing it. However there is a point at which parental incompetence triggers societal action, in the form of child protection laws. Parents must not actively harm their children emotionally or physically, neglect their children's basic needs, or endanger their children's health or well-being. The punishment for falling below this threshold can involve transfer of responsibility for the child to a guardian or removal of the child from the home.

But most parents aim for higher standards and consider it part of their job to foster growth by meeting, in addition to physical needs, a wide range of emotional and educational needs. Ethicists agree that the well-being of children requires more than maintaining bodily health, but there is little consensus regarding which of many additional needs should take precedence (Malek, 2009). Society judges parents, and parents judge themselves, based largely on the success of their children. However, there is a wide range in parental expectations in this endeavor, and there is no valid definition of either effectiveness in parenting or success in the child.

In health care, our best measurement of parental effectiveness comes from monitoring the child's growth and development, using charts and guidelines obtained from averaging the measurements of countless children. Many guidebooks provide, along with parenting advice, developmental landmarks that parents can, and often do, use to measure themselves against other parents. As the child matures, effectiveness can be measured in other ways—by the child's performance at school, or in sports, or in friendships, perhaps. All of these measures of parental effectiveness essentially compare the child to societal expectations for the successful child, with no uncontested agreement about what counts as success.

Even these weak standards cannot be applied to children who are not developing typically. We shall see that parents of children who have disabilities or complex medical problems must establish for themselves new standards for success, for their children as well as for themselves. They spend much more time in the pursuit of information that will aid in the resetting of expectations than they do acquiring the basic skills that we think of when we define caregiving.

Extreme caregiving begins, however, with the need to acquire competence in an entirely new set of caregiving skills, some of which cross into areas usually reserved for professionals. Competence from a professional caregiver is, at least in some degree, trainable and measurable. The skills and knowledge taught are centered on the science of medicine and are easily measured by exams and licensing boards. The majority of parents are not trained in medicine or nursing, nor do they need to be. Parents of children with special medical needs are offered some training in home health care nursing, usually in the last few days of hospitalization. Their skills are assessed by monitoring the child's health via frequent follow-up visits.

Competence in the practices of medicine, nursing, and other health care professions is established and assessed by the institutions that have taken responsibility for hiring and training them. According to Tronto (1993), if care is assigned to incompetent caregivers, both the inept caregiver and the organization that assigned the unqualified person to do the care are at fault. The institutions that train and assign health care providers thus take some of the responsibility to ensure care is adequate. I would argue that monitoring the child's medical progress does not complete the obligation on the part of the medical system of caring for the child in this phase. If a parent caregiver is providing inadequate care, the entirety of the blame should not fall on that parent. Some of the responsibility falls to the medical care system in which they have been assigned the task.

The burden of extreme caregiving falls on some parents at random, through accidents of genetics or disease or injury. We cannot expect to hold these parents to the same standards as we do trained health care providers, and yet we have seen the variety of professional tasks that they are routinely expected to perform. We can measure their skills in some small areas of caregiving, but we have no way of assessing overall success. We also have no real knowledge of how parents measure their own success or failure.

In this chapter, I first review the possibility of parental incompetence in extreme caregiving, using a narrative from my own experience that illustrates the many facets of competence which parents must acquire and how few options there are to correct suspected incompetence. Then I explore parents' reports of their experiences in attaining competence and how they acquired the knowledge they needed, not just to care for their children but also to ensure their success. We then explore parents' perceptions of competence: how they define it, how they acquire it, and how they evaluate themselves. We can perhaps also discover, through parent narratives, the surprisingly high standards that parents often set for themselves.

Measuring Competence

Several years ago, I received a phone call from a family physician in a tiny rural emergency room at the beginning of a long holiday weekend. The mother of a fourteen-month-old with chronic respiratory problems due to a congenital syndrome was demanding that her son be admitted to the hospital. Spencer had been born with a defect of his jaw that made it nearly impossible for him to breathe through his nose or mouth, and had eventually needed a tracheostomy. This put him at risk for respiratory problems, particularly aspiration pneumonia. He was well-known to the medical providers in the area because of his frequent respiratory illnesses.

It was pretty clear that the physician did not think that the baby was sick or, at least, any sicker than usual. His mother had taken Spencer to three different clinics that week for increasing congestion and noisy breathing. Despite her claims of worsening problems, no one had detected any obvious change in his medical condition. There had been no change in blood counts or X-rays to indicate pneumonia. But Spencer's mother thought he needed to be in the hospital, and the doctor was reluctant to refuse her. She also stated that her hospital was not equipped to care for a baby with special needs on a weekend. The hospital I was working for, in a slightly larger town thirty miles away, wasn't much bigger, but at least it had a pediatrician on call: me. I'd been hired for the week while the town's sole pediatrician was on vacation.

Already I was being called upon to make a judgment based at least partly on an estimation of competence. I did not know either the physician or the parent but could not automatically assume that the physician was correct. In my experience, mothers of chronically ill children often know when their children are seriously ill before it becomes obvious to medical providers. Sometimes even parents whose understanding of medicine is incomplete have an intimate and accurate knowledge of their own child's symptoms and reactions, which should not be ignored.

This is affirmed by several studies, including a study of mothers of chronically ill children in a large city, which found that mothers' knowledge about their child's illness, gained as part of learning to care for them, sometimes exceeded that of the people staffing small community clinics. The study reported that parents not only mastered "a wide range of knowledge" but also became "adept at getting needed attention from clinicians." They had to learn both how to follow professional advice and when to challenge it. One mother so often went against the advice of her community hospital, in favor of what she had learned at the big medical center two hours away, that the staff eventually refused to care for her daughter (Mattingly, 2014, pp. 99–100).

Another study, of parents of technology-dependent children, also found that parents were "asked to become sophisticated health care experts" and often had misunderstandings and disagreements with their child's physicians. Some of this was due to contradictory medical advice, forcing parents to choose between professionals. The parents were not always wrong, yet were "still expected to defer to, and comply with, the advice they receive from professionals." As parents gained knowledge and experience, they became more assertive, and professionals often began to either avoid them or try to pressure them into compliance with advice (Kirk, 1998, p. 111).

In Spencer's case, the family physician clearly thought that the mother was overreacting to a minor cold. She hinted that the mother might be exaggerating the illness and was seeking the opportunity to get a weekend off while her child was in the hospital. But I had no idea if the physician was equipped to recognize the subtle signs of severe illness in an infant with a tracheostomy. Three visits in one week is significant, and I felt it was time for a more extensive evaluation than could be done in a small clinic. I surprised the physician by agreeing to admit Spencer to my hospital, at least to keep an eye on him overnight.

When Spencer arrived, it was immediately obvious that things were more complicated than I'd been told. It took three people to bring him into his hospital room. His mother carried Spencer and his portable oxygen tank. His grandmother brought suction equipment and a heart monitor. A young man who turned out to be the mother's boyfriend carried a nebulizer to administer inhaled medications and two bags full of supplies, including special formula, hypoallergenic diapers, and a variety of medications not expected to be on hand at the small hospital pharmacy. The hospital indeed did not have a supply of either the formula or most of the medications.

Spencer's problems were not limited to his tracheostomy and recurrent pneumonia. After his birth, he had been transferred between several hospitals to access several different specialists. In addition to his tracheostomy, performed by an ENT surgeon, he had several bronchoscopies by a pulmonologist and had to be sent to an entirely different city for heart problems, which had required open heart surgery. No one could tell me exactly what Spencer's heart problem had been, but his mother claimed that it had been completely resolved by the surgery. Along the way, he'd been discovered to have neurological problems, including possible blindness and deafness, and severe developmental delay. He was unable to suck or swallow, so he had also needed a gastrostomy for tube feedings. He had finally gone home, to a small town that had a clinic staffed by a nurse practitioner, at five months of age. He had a tracheostomy and required frequent suctioning, a heart monitor, home oxygen, a nebulizer, and continuous gastrostomy tube feedings.

It was impossible to tell if Spencer was sick or not. He had no fever or signs of distress, and his chest X-ray, blood counts and oxygen levels were all completely normal. But he was breathing a bit rapidly, and the air passing through his trach made a gooey, congested sound. This improved after one of the nurses, against his mother's instructions, suctioned him vigorously. Tracheal suctioning is not pleasant, and Spencer cried during it. Of course, with the tracheostomy tube through his airway, he could only make desperate, gasping noises, blowing air through his tube, while tears gathered in his eyes. But it did help his noisy breathing.

During this time, the hospital staff voiced their discomfort at having to take care of this difficult case during a holiday weekend. The possibility of transferring him to a bigger hospital arose, however, I was beginning to suspect that Spencer's only problem with his breathing was that he had a cold, and his mother was reluctant to increase the frequency of suctioning. Eventually I agreed to transport him by helicopter to the nearest pediatric hospital if there was any sign of deterioration. Meanwhile, the hospital called in extra nursing and respiratory therapy staff.

Spencer's family said nothing during the negotiations which proved that a hospital with trained staff was reluctant to take on the care that they performed regularly. Trying to acknowledge this, I gestured at the surrounding commotion and said, sympathetically, "With all this, Spencer's room must look like a children's hospital." His grandmother stared at me blankly for a few seconds. "Spencer's bedroom?" she said. "He doesn't fit in the bedroom. We got him in the living room." I began to realize that the medical world that I inhabited and the world of extreme caregiving were further apart than I imagined.

Our expectation that anybody should be able to care for a child regardless of the extent of their need, raises questions within Tronto's (1993) phases of care about how we should consider competence as a moral issue. We must be careful about the assignment of blame, as we have essentially assigned random parents to an extraordinarily difficult task. We know there are many families who are not really up to competently raising a typical child, let alone coping with the multitude of responsibilities that come with extreme caregiving. Clearly, not everyone who has been assigned the tasks of extreme caregiving will be able to perform them well, particularly since there is rarely any training or preparation for them.

Children like Spencer, with multiple complex needs, are being sent home, where their parents are expected to set up miniature private hospitals and cope with any problems that might arise. Spencer's family, through no fault of their own, was not a good candidate for running a pediatric ICU. They lived in an old two-story farmhouse on the edge of a tiny town with no specialty medical care. His mother had been seventeen when

Spencer came home and had already dropped out of school. His grandmother had barely held onto her job stacking shelves at a WalMart during the months of hospitalization. When she was not at work, she helped care for Spencer. Neither Spencer's mother's boyfriend nor Spencer's father usually helped with caregiving. Yet, from a tiny living room, they were providing an extensive, time-consuming regimen, requiring some medication or procedure or task, every hour, around the clock.

A medical definition of competence in pediatric home health care can be deduced from a recent statement from the American Academy of Pediatrics that provides guidelines for clinicians who are sending a child with complex needs home from the hospital. The stated overall goal of home care is "to ensure that each child remains healthy, thrives, and obtains optimal medical home and developmental supports that promote ongoing care at home and minimize recurrent hospitalizations." Prior to discharge, the parents must be trained in use and maintenance of equipment, and taught to recognize and respond to signs of increasing illness. They also recommend that parents spend at least one or two nights at the hospital to learn all they need to know (Elias & Murphy, 2012, p. 996). Despite this, parents report that it takes about six months before they become comfortable with these technical aspects of care (Ray, 2002). Regardless of the parents' comfort levels, success at parental home care can presumably be measured at follow-up visits by tracking the child's growth and development, monitoring the effectiveness of prescribed medications, and tracking the need for medical intervention.

I imagine that the training Spencer's family received prior to going home was up to these standards, and by many measurements they were doing well. Spencer was clean and well-nourished, though the family was using a special formula of their own devising. The medical equipment they brought with them was in good working order, and they clearly knew how to use it. The mother provided a two-page list of medications, most of which she had brought with her, neatly labeled with dosage times and instructions. It took us three hours just to do the paperwork to transcribe the doses and times into the medical chart. Some of the medications were extra vitamins and skin care products that had not been prescribed by a clinician, but I saw no need to change them, since Spencer's skin looked great, including the areas around his gastrostomy and tracheostomy, which can be very difficult to keep clear.

Perhaps his mother was not doing her job of preventing illnesses and keeping him out of the hospital. She certainly was not suctioning him often enough to keep up with the congestion from his cold. I was willing to forgive her for not suctioning him often enough, since it so clearly was uncomfortable for him. I have already discussed reports that parents find it difficult to perform the dual role of parent and caregiver when uncomfortable procedures are required (Kirk et al., 2005).

At the time of admission, it was not clear if the mother's demand that her son be in the hospital was parental wisdom acquired from caregiving or a blatant attempt to get a weekend off. However, the mother and her boyfriend were not dressed for taking a child to the hospital. She was wearing a short sequined dress and heels, and he a velvet jacket and shiny black shoes. As I began the process of entering Spencer's medications into the medical record, the boyfriend announced that it was time to go. Spencer's mother left with him, clicking down the hospital corridor in her fancy heels. She never returned, though his grandmother remained at his bedside for all the hours she was not working. His condition remained stable, with no sign of anything other than a cold.

Given the difficulty of Spencer's care, I could not find much fault in using the hospital inappropriately. The family clearly needed help, and I doubted that more appropriate respite care could be found anywhere in the surrounding farmland. I found out later that the family was receiving the maximum available medical assistance, including eighteen hours a day of home health nursing. With no other expertise in the area, the family became responsible for hiring and training those workers. Unfortunately, the mother's exacting standards had driven away every trained person in the area. She was clearly not succeeding at one of the responsibilities of extreme caregiving: running a home health care agency.

More concerning to me was learning that Spencer had been to very few of his follow-up appointments. He'd seen a pulmonologist for his breathing problems, but he had not been back to see either his ENT or cardiologist. I easily compiled a list of about fifteen additional specialists that Spencer ought to be seeing; ophthalmology, audiology, dermatology, developmental pediatrics, nutrition, genetics, and physical therapy, to name a few. Unfortunately these specialists had their offices in two different cities, each over a hundred miles away, in opposite directions. The family had only one car, which belonged to his grandmother and was available only on the days on which she did not need it to drive to her job. I had no solution for this problem.

I also was disturbed that his mother did not seem terribly interested in establishing a firm diagnosis for him. No syndrome had been identified, though it was clear that Spencer's problems were global. His mother did not know if he could see or hear. Nor had she sought information about his developmental potential. In my experience, this is unusual. I have rarely met a parent whose involvement in caregiving does not include questioning every available doctor for medical information about the child's diagnosis and prognosis. We shall see that the parent narrators spend a great deal of time on this pursuit. However, the AAP guidelines for home care do not include requiring the parent to acquire medical knowledge about a child's illness, other than the technical know-how needed to provide care.

Clearly, however, Spencer's family was not in compliance with some medical recommendations. Parents who fail to appear for appointments can find themselves accused of neglect. Failure to comply with doctor's orders, regardless of the reason, is often assumed to be a sign of parental incompetence or inadequacy. If this crosses into medical neglect, the child can be removed from the parents' direct involvement. In my experience, this is both a physical and moral judgment, and carries with it the label of "bad parent." Removal of the child from the home, or even the assigning of a new guardian, is perceived as punitive by all parties involved.

Cheryl Mattingly, in a long-term anthropology study of low-income families caring for chronically ill children, noted that the penalty for perceived incompetence, or disagreement with clinicians, could be high. She states that there are "moral norms governing appropriate clinic behavior," which require mothers to participate in and follow instructions regarding their child's care. She writes,

> When clients (including family members) do not do their parts, they are labeled non-compliant. This label can have extremely serious consequences. Children can be taken out of their home and put into foster care . . . . The smallest infractions can trigger the dreaded "home visit" by a social worker to see whether he or she finds any evidence of parental neglect. (2014, p. 71)

The parents in her study viewed the clinic as a place where they were judged for their caregiving abilities, and where the price for incompetence was high.

Lia Lee, the subject of the famous book, *The Spirit Catches You and You Fall Down* (Fadiman, 1997), was actually removed from her mother's care for some months. In those years, doctors saw her mother's culture-based reluctance to give Lia seizure medications as a sign of lack of education and incompetence. In fact, Lia's seizures were extremely difficult to control. She continued having seizures in foster care, despite receiving her medications regularly, and was eventually returned home. But when she again came to the ER with unstoppable seizures, it was assumed that the mother had once again failed in her ability or willingness to administer the medications. This assumption caused her doctors to miss other possibilities, ultimately with disastrous results. This book is often studied as an example of a cultural clash but, while there are indeed cultural barriers, this sort of misunderstanding between doctor and caregiver is not unique to Hmong parents.

In Spencer's case, I called the county's Child Protection Services and learned that social workers had already done an investigation and were considering the transfer of legal guardianship to his grandmother. We knew, however, that "taking him away from his mother" in this manner would likely not facilitate access to medical care. My only option would have been transferring Spencer to one of the two big city hospitals where he'd been treated previously. If I had worded my reservations about his family's possible inadequacies strongly enough, this would have served to effectively remove him from his family's care. Spencer would spend his life in a hospital or care facility, where his mother and grandmother would have been able to visit him maybe once a week.

However, I felt that the care Spencer was receiving was loving and attentive and given to the best of the abilities of his young mother and working grandmother. While it would have been nice to accurately pinpoint his physical and developmental abilities, I also realized that these evaluations would not likely either significantly improve his outcome or simplify his care. Instead I stopped all of his nonprescription medications, added a new inhaled medication, and recommended feeding him a standard infant formula. I taught his grandmother again when, and how, to suction him, though I knew by then that her reluctance was due to kindness, not laziness or inability. I fully expected his mother to go back to his usual regimen as soon as she got him home. Likewise, I expected that the phone numbers for fifteen different specialists would go unused.

I do not know if this decision is a sign of my own incompetence. Perhaps I am a fool who let a teenage mother use my hospital as a babysitting service, without insisting that social services correct her inappropriate behavior. But I think it most likely that the care provided by his mother and grandmother was the best care that could be provided for him. I have no foreknowledge about what course might have been best for Spencer. There is no way to know whether Spencer would thrive at home without aggressive medical follow-up, or would have lived longer or better in the hospital. I do not even know what sort of outcome would either prove the validity of my trust or demonstrate his mother's (and perhaps my own) lack of competence. I will never find out. I am unlikely to see him again, and privacy laws forbid me to search for his medical records.

It is clear that there are differences in parental ability and also clear that extreme caregiving requires extreme competence in multiple areas. If we are to make moral judgments based on competence as a virtue, it would be desirable to find a balance that takes into account the difficulty of the task. I fear that no matter where we set the bar for competence, we will find parents who are unable to meet it. Yet we cannot decrease our expectation for parental capability because we lack a reasonable alternative to care for children with complex needs. Those problems lie too deeply in our medical and social systems to be resolved here, and I have no solution for them. At this point, we may be able to do nothing more than point out what has been demanded, and ask the question of whether it has become too much to expect from some, if not all, parents.

The Quest for Knowledge

Parents are usually taught the essential information they need for caregiving directly by the child's health care team and understand they must quickly learn as much as possible—to keep their children alive. Thus, the long hours involved are dictated largely by health care professionals, and parents must find a way to organize their lives in compliance with medical advice. Parents' ability to follow medical instructions and handle home medical equipment have been extensively studied in the literature, but for parents this is only the first step. The technical training is a small portion of the expertise that parents must acquire. We shall see that many parents also seek detailed and specific information about their child's health problems.

Once the child is medically stable at home, the parents' duties shift to ensuring the best long-term outcome. Parents must piece together the things they must do, from any source they can find; from special education teachers, home health care nurses, psychologists, speech and occupational therapists, developmental specialists, other parents, and, of course, a multitude of physicians (Elias & Murphy, 2012). For many, this requires a deep understanding of their child's medical problems, as well as knowledge of their child as a unique individual with a unique way of expressing those problems.

Neither the knowledge they acquire to accomplish this task nor what they think about their newfound abilities have been studied. Since competence is a moral value desired in parent caregivers, I believe it is important to understand from the parents themselves how they acquire information and frame their competence.

One of the first things that becomes apparent in parent memoirs is how little attention is devoted to the act of caregiving even in books that describe the experience of extreme caregivers. In *The Boy in the Moon* (2011), Ian Brown spends the first chapter describing the difficulties encountered in a night as primary caregiver for his son Walker, but then rarely mentions it again. The endless round of sleepless nights, messy feedings, and diaper changes thereafter becomes a background thread acknowledged only by infrequent reminders of fatigue. Some of the narrators, such as Josh Greenfeld in *A Child Called Noah* (1970) or Charles Hart in *Without Reason* (1989) never mention this aspect of care at all, though both of their sons surely must have had feeding and diapering issues. Whether this is because their wives were doing the majority of this sort of care, or whether this earlier generation did not talk about such things, is unclear.

When caregiving is mentioned, it is usually in the form of confession of inadequacy, often tinged with humor. Ian Brown speaks of the "Gobi desert" that the carpet beneath his son's bed has become because of the many times that he has disconnected Walker's G-tube improperly and spilled formula on the floor. For him, the technology is just there and using it is a complicated but necessary ingredient in the goal of getting through the night. Charles Hart disparagingly refers to his caregiving duties as becoming a "house husband," something he does not seem particularly proud of. The only description he gives of his caregiving duties is to say that he has become "the primary homemaker, chauffeur, and resident child development specialist" (1989, p. 158).

Instead of concentrating on the details of their caregiving, all the authors seem much more interested in acquiring medical information so they can understand what they are doing. In my experience, parents are similarly eager for medical knowledge. The exception is the mother and grandmother of Spencer, stranded in a small town without access to specialized care. It is unusual for a parent to be unable to name with exactitude a heart defect that required major surgery. Many can draw the diagram of the heart problem from memory. It is also unusual for a parent whose child clearly has multiple disabilities to be uninterested in identifying a syndrome or pursuing a more accurate diagnosis. Spencer was still quite young, though. It is likely that his mother was merely overwhelmed, and had no time for questions, or access to those who might answer them.

One mother of a child with Down syndrome likened the birth of her son to being unexpectedly and unwillingly enrolled in college. In an essay titled "The School of Life," she describes the classes that she must now attend. After "Expectations 101" and "Appearances 101," the courses in which she mourns the loss of a typical family, she is rapidly enrolled in "Health 105." She writes,

> Since children born with Down syndrome are more likely to have special health concerns, I learned about the many medical problems my son could have. I studied diagrams of the human heart. I made mental notes about the symptoms of leukemia. I learned what an otolaryngologist is and how to spell "ophthalmologist." There was a long chapter on genetics and reproduction. (Bremer, 2007, p. 88)

Later, when her son is diagnosed with leukemia, she is enrolled in "Health 201" and "Chemotherapy 501," a very advanced class. She recalls that she "felt sorry for the parents [she] met of typical kids with cancer because they hadn't completed any of the preliminary coursework" (p. 89). Parents faced with a child's illness will begin, to the best of their ability, to acquire medical knowledge. That knowledge becomes an integral part of caregiving.

Several of the parent narrators use the metaphor of a life journey, or a quest, to describe, not their caregiving, but the acquisition of knowledge. At least two narrators use the word "journey" in the subtitles of their books: Greenfeld's book is *A Child Called Noah: A Family Journey* (1970), and Brown's full title is *The Boy in the Moon: A Father's Journey to Understand His Extraordinary Son* (2011). That journey is largely a quest for medical knowledge, with the hope of understanding what is happening to their child, and themselves. Almost all parent memoirs, even the ones without the word journey in their titles, spend many pages describing their pursuit of understanding, beginning with investigations into the science of medicine. Their search for medical knowledge can be seen as the way in which parents train themselves, after the fact and out of necessity, to be competent caregivers. They frequently express dissatisfaction with their abilities, implying that competence in caregiving demands more from them than the ability to perform physical care.

We measure the competence of clinicians by testing their medical knowledge, usually after a period of intense training. Unlike professional caregivers, parents begin their "training" after the need for it has arrived. There is no decision to undertake caregiving as a career and no prior experience. For parents, there is also no test at the end, nor, in fact, any defined standard of success or endpoint to the learning process. But the quest for medical information runs as a thread through parent narratives, as promising new diagnoses or therapies are discovered, attempted and, often, discarded. Perhaps this is the realm where parents find their identity as competent caregivers?

To test this premise, I first looked at the parents' journeys for information, to find out how they conducted their searches and how they felt about the information they received. I found an unexpectedly high level of knowledge that, since it is rarely recognized, I wish to emphasize. I also found that parents do not actually consider this knowledge as a form of expertise and instead defer to physicians and other scientific experts.

The Search for Information

The various parent narrators all speak of extensively researching their child's medical problems, using the most recent diagnosis or professional recommendations as a launching point. Many of them seek second opinions, often finding and arranging visits with a variety of specialists on their own. They seek specific information about their child's diagnosis and promising new therapies from professional journals and books. In the past they sometimes had to resort to medical textbooks for explanations of unfamiliar concepts; now, of course, they use the internet. They also gather advice from teachers, therapists, and even other parents, particularly from parent support groups and websites.

The journey begins either with the arrival of a medical diagnosis or with the realization that a diagnosis is needed. Some parents receive a diagnosis prenatally through genetic screening and begin their quest for knowledge prior to birth. Sometimes parents are given a firm diagnosis or name of a syndrome shortly after birth. Others, such as the parents of extremely premature infants, endure a time of limbo in the hospital where diagnosis, or even survival, is in question. For many more, particularly the parents of children with autism or delayed development, the search begins at home with a dawning recognition that the child is not developing typically. Coming to terms with a diagnosis can be a slow process, which is complicated by the need to grieve for the expected child and accept the child who has actually arrived. Acceptance is often accomplished after detailed research into the child's diagnosis and aided (or sometimes hindered) by understanding the child's medical problems.

Almost all the parents contributing to the essay collection *Gifts: Mothers Reflect on How Children with Down Syndrome Enrich Their Lives* (Soper,

2007) are initially devastated by the diagnosis. They reach the point of acceptance through consultation with medical professionals and by reading medical textbooks or manuals about Down syndrome. Many of the contributors found that the information available from these was often negative and sought other sources. One of the stated goals of the book is to speak from the other side of that initial dark journey. The editor states, "Given the fear and dread that commonly surround a diagnosis of Down syndrome, it's clear that these uplifting voices need to be heard by the world—and especially the parents facing this diagnosis for their child" (Soper, p. xxiii).

But not all parents are provided a firm diagnosis early in the process. Their search begins with the need to establish a diagnosis; to find out what, if anything, is wrong with their child. This is a frustratingly gradual process, often lasting for months or even years. It is not unusual for diagnoses to be made and then discarded, as the journey of discovery progresses. For many the journey is literal, as they travel to cities with pediatric centers for a series of consultations with specialists.

The desire to find a medical answer for the problem, in the early stages, is often balanced by a hope that there really isn't anything wrong. The acquisition of any diagnosis, even a wrong one, at once dashes hopes of normalcy and provides a new avenue for research. This voyage of discovery is an integral part of parent narratives, taking up a good deal of pages and becoming the main narrative arc of many memoirs.

Once a diagnosis is proposed, it becomes a focus for research about the disease process and a search for medical treatments or therapy. If the diagnosis is uncertain, parents might research alternative explanations in the hope of finding a curable or less frightening possibility. If the diagnosis is known, they might hope to discover a new cure or perhaps a lesser known and more effective treatment. They also often wish to understand what they might have done that has caused their child's problems, though we have seen that the guilt parents feel is not based on reason and is very difficult to assuage.

The advancement of medical knowledge has, perhaps, refined parents' searches, but it has not made them less difficult. It is surprising how similar the journey is compared with times past. In 1970, when Greenfeld began a journey to discover what was wrong with his son, Noah, autism was an obscure problem. Some of the information he sought so eagerly and travelled so far to obtain is now readily available, as autism has become a more common diagnosis. Now, a parent who learns that her child has autism does not need years to investigate what this means, as Greenfeld did. But though there are differences in the way autism is diagnosed and perceived today, the journey to discover what autism means for a modern family will in many ways be similar to that of Greenfeld's. Advances in medical knowledge, while significant, have not arrived at the answers parents desire. No one can accurately predict, particularly in the early years, how autism will affect a child's future. There are more definitive treatments, but nothing guaranteed, and there is certainly nothing that explains why some children are affected and others are not.

For less common diagnoses, medical science is still struggling along with the parents. Ian Brown's (2011) son, Walker, born in 1996, received his diagnosis of CFC (Cardiofaciocutaneous syndrome) in 1997, when he was eight months old—an extraordinarily early age. The Browns had the advantage of living near a major pediatric center, and their pediatrician had an interest in unusual syndromes. Brown reports that CFC was first described in 1979, and there were only about forty reported cases worldwide at the time of Walker's diagnosis. Brown writes, "The medical profession—at least the handful of doctors who studied cardiofaciocutaneous syndrome, or knew what it was—was learning about the syndrome as we did" (Brown, 2011, pp. 7–8). Twenty years later, a parent learning about CFC will find little increase in professional knowledge or awareness.

As they conduct their search, parents also have to gain a familiarity with the mysterious language of medicine: the words used by professionals to describe medical symptoms and conditions. Many of the narrators provide the exact Latin descriptions of their child's problems or diagnoses, carefully explaining the meaning of those words for the uninitiated reader. Some rattle off lists of terms, effectively reproducing for the reader the confusion caused by their number and complexity. One parent (Bremer, 2007) even provides a list of the three-letter acronyms she learned, fifteen of them in all, without explanation or translation, as if to emphasize the seeming impossibility of them all.

Ian Brown discusses his reactions to the use of medical language on several occasions. He seems impressed by the usefulness and the exactitude of their meanings, but sometimes he seems overwhelmed by them. The words invoke for him a science-fictional attitude that he finds at once impressive and unrealistic. After casually listing the names of thirteen of Walker's medications, he writes, "They sounded like the names of ambassadors to an intergalactic conference of aliens" (2011, p. 45). His reaction to the acronyms used in genetic research is similar: "The genes and their complicated acronyms (most of which related to their chemical composition) sounded like newly discovered planets to me, as baffling and rarefied as genetics itself" (p. 166).

Sometimes the precision of those words is comforting. Talking about an early visit to his pediatrician, Brown notices a multitude of unfamiliar words on his son's chart. He lists many of them for the reader, offering short translations in parentheses. They are mostly Latin descriptions of Walker's facial features, as he finds out later, but the doctor's knowledge of them is both reassuring and daunting. The pediatrician, he writes, "always used the scientific terms on the boy's chart—it made for more accurate communication with other doctors. They were serious words, embodying a professional standard of exactitude." Yet even as he praises them, Brown is wary of them. He continues, "But Walker Brown was a hard boy to be exact about" (p. 28).

Charles Hart also found medical language reassuring at times, reporting being impressed and comforted by some of the labels eventually attached to his son Ted. One of Ted's unusual behaviors was a tendency to repeat things he'd heard, without seeming to be aware of their meanings. After seeing an expert in communication disorders, Hart says, "The doctor . . . taught us the technical terms for the senseless language we heard so often: 'echolalia' for the repeated phrases of other's speech and 'idioglossia,' meaning language of idiots, for Ted's original but nonsensical phrases" (1989, p. 66). Even though Hart realizes that the Latin word is merely a description of the problem, and not terribly complimentary to Ted, the use of the word idioglossia made it into an identifiable symptom, and therefore more impressive and accurate.

The words used as diagnostic labels are particularly difficult, as they create both hope and anxiety in parents. A diagnosis means that a problem has been identified and pinpointed, which leads to the possibility of a cure. But for a parent on a journey to discover what, if anything, is wrong, a diagnosis means that a problem exists. During the phase where Noah's diagnosis is still uncertain, Greenfeld expresses his reluctance at times to visit specialists; "I'm afraid to go to a doctor because I know that we'll then find out whatever the specialist knows. Expertise discovers itself in its subjects" (1970, p. 51). As long as Noah remains without an exact diagnosis, Greenfeld can hope that he will just outgrow his problems.

Brown echoes this sentiment with his feelings about his first referral to a genetics specialist; "Any parent of a child with a syndrome remembers the day he or she is told to see the genetics department. It is the second circle of diagnostic hell. What has been, to that point, a matter of health, something you could fix, is suddenly a matter of science, carved in genetic stone" (2011, p. 31). The diagnosis seems to nail down the problem, and make it true and real, in a way that physical descriptions, even in Latin, do not.

The words of a diagnosis can also be used to obscure problems. An example of this is Ted Hart's diagnosis of pervasive developmental disorder (PDD), which he was given at age five. Reading about his diagnosis as a pediatrician, and knowing that this was at the time a newly accepted way of describing autism, I thought that the doctors had finally (at last!) arrived at the correct diagnosis, which was clear to me from Hart's descriptions of Ted's problems. But Hart did not know this. It was two years before he learned the meaning of those words, when he recognized his son's symptoms on an autism checklist. When confronted with this, Hart's doctor admitted to using the new term deliberately to obscure the more well-known, and presumed to be more horrifying, diagnosis of autism (Hart, 1989, pp. 75–76).

Parents will encounter shifts in diagnostic terms as new phrases are developed that more accurately depict current medical thinking or that have not yet been associated with stigmatized problems. For example, phrases like "emotionally disturbed" and "childhood psychosis" have been replaced by more accurate concepts such as "sensory integration disorder" or "hypersensitivity to stimuli." These terms have all been used, over the years, to describe similar symptoms usually attributed to autism, but they have very different diagnostic implications and social resonance. I expect that these diagnostic terms will continue to shift, as science refines our understanding of autism, and as people inevitably begin to use older terms in a negative context.

Even though autism is more accepted today, some parents still wish to avoid the term by using carefully selected words. Another author of a narrative about a child with special needs, Priscilla Gilman, in *The Anti-Romantic Child* (2011), uses the language of medicine to disguise her child's diagnosis from both the reader and herself. She reports that she is repelled by the language of medicine, saying, "There is nothing less romantic, literary, or lyrical than the language of pathology, diagnosis, symptom checklists" (p. 100). Her son Benjamin's diagnosis, she reports, is hyperlexia with sensory integration dysfunction. This is a modern description of some of the symptoms on the autism spectrum, much like Ted Hart's diagnosis of pervasive developmental disorder. Perhaps because Benjamin is not as severely affected as Ted, his mother prefers this lyrical collection of words over the simpler diagnosis of autism. It sets Benjamin apart and clouds the exact nature of her son's problems.

The medical words inspire both confidence and humility, and a parent who has been through the diagnostic process learns to both hope for and distrust them. Ian Brown summarizes the complexity of this in his own beautifully complex language. He has listed, in italics and without defining them, some thirty medical terms that have been applied to Walker in association with his diagnosis of CFC. For Brown, these terms have a deep significance. "The language of Walker's strangeness held me captive," he writes.

> New words had been invented for a new creation, infused with the pretend exactitude of scientific nomenclature, as if all the labels said something helpful and useful, which of course in any comparative sense they did. The alluring multisyllabic complexity necessary to describe a simpleton, to use the old, once-scientific word for such a boy. (2011, p. 158)

He is held captive by the brilliant words but at the same time recognizes their essential meaninglessness. Years of impressive-sounding scientific progress is relegated to nothing except different words to describe a child whose problems can't be solved. And yet perhaps there is still a tiny hope that, in a comparative sense, some progress has been, and yet will be, made.

All the parents eventually learn that a diagnosis only gives a name to the problem; it does not solve it. Nor does it entirely define the extent of the problem, since even the most well-established diagnosis encompasses a large amount of individual variability. From a parent's perspective, the words used to identify a problem are never adequate. They cannot tell the parent the things they most dearly want to know: how the child's future might differ from that of the typical child they had expected; how they can provide for the child the best life possible; and, most importantly, who the child is. (We will return in Chapter 7 to the question of diagnosis and the child's identity.)

With their seeming importance and almost deliberate incomprehensibility, these words inspire confidence in the scientific ability and professionalism of the person who can use them easily. However, the words also serve, by emphasizing a knowledge base that is not generally accessible, to humble the layperson and point out how little he knows. The language of medicine creates a distance between parent and professional, and emphasizes to the layperson that they are not trained in all the intricacies of science, that their knowledge is limited. The parents who become extreme caregivers must dwell in a prolonged and often discouraging intimacy with medical providers, who often dictate the care they must perform. Perhaps a lack of fluency in medicine's obscure language contributes to feelings of inadequacy parents might harbor. The language of medicine holds unexpected power, and clinicians would do well to wield its words carefully.

Level of Knowledge Attained

In my experience as a pediatrician, I have met parents of children with a variety of medical problems who demonstrate considerable medical knowledge and seem hungry for more. I have never tested any parent on their level of their knowledge, of course, but most parents absorbed any information I was able to give them. Neither the level of information that parents attain in caring for a child with special needs, nor their understanding of that information, has been systematically studied. As I read the parent narratives, I was able to evaluate the medical data the authors presented, and I found the accuracy and depth of their knowledge to be surprisingly high. More surprising to me, though, was how little parents regarded their competence in this regard.

Memoirs written by the parents of preemies document the rapid acquisition of expertise in the common problems of prematurity and their consequences. In her recollection of events, Deanna Fei, the mother of a micro-preemie, provides not only the severity of her daughter's intraventricular hemorrhage but also the medical information on which that diagnosis was based. She describes the appearance of her daughter's cranial ultrasound and reports the current statistics for its likelihood and possible outcomes (2015, p. 113). Vicky Forman provides an accurate, detailed description of Retinopathy of Prematurity, or ROP, the technical name for the damage to the eye caused by exposure to high oxygen in premature infants, that was the cause of her premature son's blindness. She gives detailed descriptions of the zones and stages of ROP, along with the treatment that might be required for each one (2009, p 88).

Parents of children with Down syndrome are likewise well-informed. Michael Berube's book about his son with Down syndrome, *Life As We Know It: A Father, a Family, and an Exceptional Child* (1996), reveals the in-depth research its author performed. His discussion of Down syndrome starts with the process of mitosis and ends many pages later with theories of "difference" based on genetics (pp. 17–24). He writes, "I got hold of everything within reach on genetics, reproduction, and 'abnormal' human development" (p 14). He does not limit his research to medicine. His search to understand Down syndrome wanders through Wittgenstein's theories of language acquisition, Foucault and disability studies, and the history of the popular music his son had come to love.

Emily Rapp also journeyed into unexpected realms to care for her dying son. Rapp studied the meaning of life, and when to let go of it. She studied grief with the same precision and attention to detail that other parents study the literature about Down syndrome or CFC. She learned to live, she writes,

> a life of heightened presence and constant mourning, an activity of which I became a scientist. Each day I picked apart my grief with a little knife; I combed through it; I boiled it in petri dishes and tried to blow it up. I sprinkled it with gas and lit a match, watched it burn, put out the fire. It always came back . . . (2013, p. 177)

To study grief, she studied medicine, philosophy, religious texts, the poetry of Dana Levin, and Joan Didion's memoir on loss, *The Year of Magical Thinking*.

Ian Brown's descriptions of the advances in genetics and behavioral neurology are precisely written and full of up-to-date information, some of which is on a frontier of medicine of which I, as a pediatrician, am only vaguely aware. Based on his intricate description of CFC, I contacted the mother of Savannah, the young woman we met at the beginning of this book, who had been my patient for a few years before moving out of state. Despite seeing numerous specialists at our pediatric hospital after her birth in 2004, Savannah's illness had remained a mystery. It seemed to me that CFC might be our long-sought diagnosis. Her mother was way ahead of me. Savannah was then eighteen and was being followed by specialists at another major pediatric center. Geneticists there had given her a working diagnosis of CFC, though she had not tested positive for any of the genetic markers so far identified.

Ian Brown found websites dedicated to CFC and related syndromes where, along with advice and sympathy, parents swap information on the latest discoveries. He considers many of these parents experts in the field. In his opinion, some of the mothers in this CFC network, "knew more than any doctor, and were widely consulted for medical and technical help" (2011, p. 135). In the course of his travels to study CFC, Brown met two mothers who had discovered the existence of CFC on their own. They had brought journal articles and photographs to their pediatricians for verification, an act not always appreciated. Both of those children were eventually confirmed as CFC by genetic testing. Brown concludes, after interviewing a number of other CFC parents, "Most parents of CFC children know more about the affliction than their pediatricians" (p. 9). I think he is correct in this assessment and that this is true for many syndromes, both common and rare.

Despite their up-to-date, accurate knowledge, however, parent narrators rarely claim any sort of expertise for themselves. They are more likely, instead, to report their inadequacies. Meanwhile, they receive information and advice from professionals with a humble deference, seeming to assume that professional knowledge is superior to their own.

I suspect that Josh Greenfeld, after reading medical books about brain damage and "mental retardation," emotional disturbances, and patterning, actually knew as much or more than any of the doctors who saw his son Noah. Yet he calls his knowledge "my amateur diagnostic attempts" (1970, p. 69), and disparagingly reports that he changes his ideas about Noah's diagnosis based on whatever book he is reading at the time. As he gains more knowledge, he becomes less trusting of Noah's doctors, saying things like, "Parents will find themselves getting little in the way of help and much in the way of confusion from the medical profession" (p. 5). But he continues to contact new professionals with hope based on respect. For example, he describes Dr. Ivar Lovass, one of the pioneers of a treatment for autism then called "operant conditioning," as "a virtuoso therapist," who can " 'play the patient' with the skill of a classically trained musician hip to all the joys of jazz improvisation" (p. 145).

Decades later, Portia Iversen, founder of Cure Autism Now and mother of a son with autism, also reports reading a massive amount of scientific literature, including acquiring a tutor for herself in basic sciences and molecular biology. She gives herself the highest praise I found expressed in any parent memoir, "I had become well versed in matters of science" (2006, p. 39). Her praise for physicians and scientists is much higher, however. "I was in awe," she says of one scientist who was, she reports, "delving ever deeper into the unknowable core of consciousness" (p. 60). Like Greenfeld, she met Ivar Lovass, who by then had changed the name of his techniques to "applied behavioral analysis." In preparation, she "made sure he knew that I'd read every research paper he'd ever written, except for the first few which I could not find." His response is merely to provide her with those unavailable papers. "I felt honored," she says (p. 27). Later, before witnessing neuropsychologic testing, she says, "Nor could I even imagine those highly complicated tests they called psychophysics tests, which only experts in neuroscience and psychology could administer, analyze, and understand" (p. 151). Yet she describes, accurately and without apparent irony, possibilities for understanding autism that those eminent neuropsychologists frequently seem to miss.

Ian Brown also belittles his extensive research into CFC saying, "I worked at home on the dining room table, plowing my way through incomprehensible papers on genetics or neurology" (2011, p. 51). He then provides a brief but precise description of one of the papers he's been reading, a complicated theory about the connection between nerve myelinization and out-of-control behavior. Brown is much more impressed with Walker's pediatrician's efforts, whom he imagines as, "leafing through the medical literature on rare afflictions" and "trying to find a particular plant in a vast garden of exotic flowers, each one more bizarre than the next" (p. 30). I have already praised Brown's accuracy and thoroughness in describing his son's condition, but, although he describes other parents as experts, he never claims this for himself.

Vicky Forman likewise does not recognize her expertise. By the time her son receives a diagnosis of infantile spasms, a particularly disturbing type of seizures, she has suspected the diagnosis for some days and already read the medical literature about it, including learning about treatment with vigabitrin, a drug that was still considered experimental. Her father, a physician, accompanies her to the neurology visit where the diagnosis is finally pronounced. He admits that he, too, suspected the diagnosis from Forman's description of the seizures. Forman seems not to recognize the level of knowledge she had obtained from her "desperate weekend of research," but she refers to her father as a "terrific diagnostician" whose ability to diagnose her son "elevated him to the role of psychic" (2009, pp. 182–183). Her son indeed was able to enter a trial for vigabitrin, though he was unfortunately not a responder to it.

A few parents were actively discouraged from seeking medical knowledge from other physicians. Ted Hart's parents approached their primary physician with a request for a second opinion, on the advice of one of Ted's preschool teachers, who didn't feel comfortable with his current diagnosis of "mental retardation." Hart writes, "Our pediatrician scoffed at getting a second opinion. He implied that we were emotionally immature for failing to accept the first opinion and threatened that he would no longer see Ted as a patient if we continued to discuss his condition with 'people on the street' " (1989, pp. 58–59). The physician's disparagement, not just of Hart, but of all nonphysician expertise is plain. Years later Hart blamed himself for failing to diagnose autism from a behavior checklist available since 1943. "[H]ow could I, with my education and community contacts, have remained ignorant for so long, never knowing that my brother's and son's problems could be explained by a disorder others had named and studied?" (p. 71). His son's doctor had hidden the diagnosis deliberately, but Hart still blamed himself rather that the doctor for the oversight.

Some clinicians regarded parents' tendency to pursue high-level medical information as a form of denial or a sign of parents' inability to come to terms with a difficult diagnosis. While his son was still in the hospital after being diagnosed with Down syndrome, Michael Berube and his wife began studying genetics textbooks. He reports,

> At one point a staff nurse was sent in to check on *our* mental health, and she found us babbling about meiosis and monoploids, wondering anew that Jamie had "gotten" Down syndrome the second he became a zygote. When the nurse inadvertently left behind her notes, Janet sneaked a peek. "Parents seem to be intellectualizing," she read. (1996, p. 14)

The nurse was hinting that the Berubes were using the acquisition of information to hide from the reality of the diagnosis. They seemed to be aware that the term "intellectualizing" was not exactly complimentary, but, rather than be offended by this, Berube decided to claim it; "Parents seem to be intellectualizing," he repeats, "And why not?" (p. 24).

These incidents are all fairly minor discouragements of parents' search for knowledge. For the most part, the professional world rarely actively prevents these parent-authors from trying to inform themselves as best as they can. However, no parent's memoir reveals an example of the opposite occurring: of medical professionals encouraging parents to gain a deeper understanding of what their child faces. No one reported being congratulated or affirmed in their astuteness by a medical professional. Mostly their knowledge was either vaguely belittled or ignored.

Despite the vast amount of research they have done and the extensive knowledge they have obtained, none of these authors ever claims any kind of expertise or clinical competence. Though they have become something like experts on their child's individual illnesses, often surpassing the knowledge of general doctors, they don't ever claim this as a valuable skill, or an acquiring of competence. While they might praise the abilities of other parents, the words they use to describe their own acquisition of knowledge are often quite disparaging. In contrast, they frequently offer glowing descriptions of the competence of the various professionals with whom they interact. They consider themselves, at best, barely competent amateurs.

In a care ethic that defines good caregiving in terms of competence, it is disturbing to me that such expertise is discounted by the person acquiring it as a part of caregiving. The lack of recognition of medical knowledge suggests to me that we, as professionals, are not providing as much support as we could. For the many parents who dive into medicine as part of their journey with their child, a significant part of their life work is going unrecognized.

I do not mean to suggest that medical knowledge should be used to judge the competence of parents. We cannot expect every parent to become a medical expert. But if this way of acquiring competence is not visible, even to the people doing it, they lose one measure by which many caregivers are succeeding brilliantly.

I have met parents whose knowledge is extensive and very helpful. I have also met parents who have formed mistaken ideas about medicine. There is not enough data to compare the relative frequency with which information acquired by parents is actually useful as opposed to incorrect. However, I would be inclined to respect parents' knowledge unless there is actual data showing that what they believe might be harmful to their child.

If there is new information on cause, diagnosis, or treatment of any chronic disabling pediatric problem, it is likely that some parents will find out about it well before their pediatricians. It would be wise to pay attention to what is learned through parent networks and to, at least, read any paper that might be offered for our consideration. I recommend that clinicians actively listen to any theories or information parents bring forward. I would not hesitate to provide textbooks or journal articles that might help parents in their research. The rapport developed with a parent who is treated as an equal in a scientific endeavor can be invaluable.

Facing Failure

A few years ago, I was catching up, by a long-distance phone call, with a friend whose son has severe autism. Sandy has dealt with a series of medical crises, during the decades I have known her, by gathering as much information as possible. As soon as Jack was diagnosed, she began studying autism, attending seminars, and participating in parent support groups. She quickly became an expert in the field, giving her own lectures and becoming an area consultant in autism. Her occasional help, suggesting new therapies or informing me about emerging theories about the cause of autism, has been invaluable in my pediatric practice. She knew far more about the brain science of autism and the current promising therapies than I did, though she always dismissed this comparison of her own knowledge to my own. But that day, she had an exciting new breakthrough to report.

"Guess what we learned! Guess what Jack can do now," she demanded, proudly. Then, without waiting for an answer, she announced, "We learned to poop in the bathroom!"

Jack, at age twelve, was nonverbal and not yet toilet trained. He had, up to that point, been using hidden corners of the house to do his business. And now Sandy had successfully taught him to use the bathroom. "We" hadn't yet learned to actually use the toilet, but at least the surprises were limited now to a single, appropriate room. At the time, I was appalled, rather than impressed. I understood the importance of this step, but could not think about it from her perspective. I did not realize that this was a statement of competence as, or possibly more, important than any new fact she learned about the science of autism. It was a triumph for both Jack and Sandy, and I could not properly recognize or celebrate it.

I have said that success in parenting is measured, by both parents and society, by observing the success of their children. Parents find competence (and bragging rights) in comparing their children with standard developmental milestones or measurements of success provided by guidebooks. But these guidelines are incorrect when applied to children with disabilities. This is particularly true for children with intellectual disabilities, since many of our scales depend on mastering certain types of learning at school.

Because of the increased level of dependency, and the unpredictable delays in expected developmental stages, learning both at school and at home is a uniquely different path for each individual child. For all extreme caregiving parents, new goals and new expectations, ones that match their children's level of ability, must be set, in an ever-changing discovery of new standards for success. Each child's individual progress is different, with different milestones to be celebrated. Since there is no gauge to measure the developmental progress that is made, one difficult day at a time, this often involves reassessing and setting new parameters for reaching ordinary goals.

But adjusting to new expectations is not an easy task for many parents. Ian Brown writes, "I was convinced we were alone. It's hard to explain how we felt for having failed to teach Walker to sleep or speak or eat or pee or even look at us—can you imagine the magnitude of that failure? I know it is not rational, but we felt responsible" (2011, p. 225). And Greenfeld, in a later book written when Noah was a teenager, says, "I guess I am always hypertense when Noah is home. He reminds me that he is an insoluble problem, a metaphysical math course that I am forever flunking" (1986, p. 324). The sense of failure runs deep in both of their memoirs.

Ian Brown (2011) uses an extended description of his son Walker's toys to express his own sense of failure. Over the years, various developmental experts have brought to their home a collection of special toys that were supposed to stimulate Walker's development. Many of them had been lent or rented from now-forgotten sources, left behind in the hope that Walker might learn something from them, though Brown remains confused as to exactly what that lesson might have been. Walker never responded to any of them. They lie in abandoned heaps around his house, bright with hope and stamped with mysterious instructions that hint at success, a reminder of all the expertise that has been invested in Walker. But at the same time, they are just toys, ridiculous objects from which to expect so much.

Yet, even while he is making fun of their essential silliness and inexplicable purpose, Brown seems to accept that it was his own inabilities—not understanding the toys, or not using them often enough, or not forcing them on Walker—that caused Walker's lack of response. He also takes their continued presence in his home as a sign of a different sort of incompetence. Most of them were supposedly loans, to be returned someday to the company or program that provided them. That he has never had the time or energy to accomplish this bothers Brown, as does the fact that he has now forgotten where most of them came from. He will never be able to return them and, since they are not his, he will never be able to throw them out. So they persist as a reminder of both failures, the incompetence of disorganization and the larger failure to help his son (pp. 18–23).

This sense of failure is part of the narrative arc of their stories. These are not narratives of redemption with triumph over disease at the end. They are quest narratives in which parents embark on a journey to understand their children and themselves, informed by the discovery of medical knowledge. They do find small triumphs along the way, but ultimately these narrators become disillusioned with medicine, and themselves, when they fail to make a significant difference in their child's progress. Their disappointment in the broken promise of science is often expressed as a personal failure.

It will come as no surprise that parents, particularly those whose children require prolonged and only partially successful medical treatment, can become disillusioned with the promise of medicine. Ian Brown provides perhaps the best description of this. He sums up his many visits to the children's hospital, each one holding hope and frustration and despair, writing:

> All those stuffed animals in the hospital store in the lobby of the brilliant children's hospital in the middle of the downtown of the brilliant genius city! And yet the place was filled with doctors who couldn't help my boy. I developed a degree of skepticism toward the medical profession that tended to show itself after the fourth doctor in a row told me something I already knew. . . I learned an almost geological patience. (2011, p. 63)

I found a similar message deep within a video game called "That Dragon, Cancer." The game was written by the parents of an infant who had died of brain cancer. Their game design included anonymous cards, drawings, and letters from other families buried in the landscape. I found this one floating in the water next to an abandoned life preserver:

> I am at [a children's hospital], and nobody wants to be here. Even as an internationally recognized temple of healing every inch of it is terror . . .. There is art on the walls and rooms which is designed to evoke a jungle of some kind, and I resent it. Every giraffe is my sworn enemy. (Green et al., 2015)

These two messages, from divergent sources, express a similar deep frustration and anger at medicine that seems to center on the bright, hopeful decor used to supposedly comfort children and their parents. They also hint at a sense of personal failure at the narrator's inability to put aside resentment and join in the hopeful, helpful celebration of medicine.

There is a deeper reason behind many of the narrators' feelings of resentment and failure however. Those parents whose children remain nonverbal begin to look to science to understand their child. Though the stated reason for undertaking the search for knowledge is often expressed in the possibility of benefit for their child, the ultimate wish of many parents is to know who their child is, and what he might say to them, if he could. One way to do this is to try to understand the changes in the child's body brought about by their medical condition. Ian Brown describes his journey into medicine:

> I was always looking for a context in which to make sense of Walker, in which his disorganized life (and my unavoidable devotion to it) might take on more meaning and purpose . . .. What I had yet to find out was *why* he

was the way he was. And so I turned to science, to see if the laboratory could explain my boy Walker. (2011, pp. 156–157)

He approaches science, particularly genetics, in hopes that it might hold, at least, an explanation of Walker's life. He knows that he will not really discover the meaning of life in Walker's DNA, but he is desperate to close the distance between himself and his son. Even though his travels to visit specialists and genetics laboratories often move him physically away from Walker, he calls his search, "work[ing] my way closer to Walker" (p. 112). Everything he learns about his son's diagnosis seems to have the potential to increase his understanding both of Walker and of himself.

Brown's quest for scientific knowledge is deeply tied to an attempt to discover Walker's inner self. When he finds out that three genes associated with CFC have been found, he worries that the discovery will change Walker for him, change the private and odd relationship they have developed. It takes over a year for the test to become available, and for the Canadian medical system to agree to do it. By the time the test is done, Brown is aware that it will change nothing for him or for Walker, that, in fact, the test itself might be an intrusion:

> To test, or not to test: that is the question. Whether 'tis calmer in the mind to ignore the touts and dreams of genetic research, or to scan each cracked gene known to man, and by testing think we have an answer. To test and test and test some more, and by this test pretend it ends the heartache and the thousand natural shocks his small flesh is heir to. 'Tis a consummation devoutly to be wished! (2011, p. 169)

Medical science holds no answers, no effective channel to Walker, yet it is the only place to look. Brown never quite convinces himself that medicine does not hold some key to unlock Walker's mind. But no one will be able to understand Walker better than Brown himself, and Brown is unable to reach him.

Charles Hart (1989) expresses his doubts directly. "We also felt a sense of failure," he recalls. "In spite of the years of family counseling and our growing expertise in autism, we felt incompetent that we couldn't apply this knowledge more effectively. Understanding Ted's disability didn't enable us to direct his behavior in a positive way" (p. 215). No matter what Charles learned, Ted remained beyond his reach, unable to communicate his frustrations and deeper feelings verbally. All this knowledge, this medical competence, while it was helpful at times, was never sufficient to meet this goal of understanding his son.

Walker and Ted remain unable to communicate despite multiple therapies. Their fathers become competent in the science of medicine, but it is not enough to reach their sons. Despite the inability of medical science to provide answers, they always takes the weight of that failure back on themselves. Their sense of failure arises, I believe, not from the lack of acknowledgement of their own expertise, but from the fact that medical information, once obtained, does not provide the answers they need. They are still unable to communicate with their child; unable to determine their unique desires, discover what they might be thinking, and understand who they are.

I suspect that the sense of failure expressed by these narrators is not unusual. These authors' search for knowledge about their child's condition is to them an essential task. Their new knowledge is integrated deeply into their lives, as new therapies become part of the daily routine of care. It changes how they think about their child and themselves. They use their knowledge to better the child's life and ensure the most promising future available. They want to know who their child is, and who he might become, even if the opportunities for becoming are limited.

The disappointment in themselves and their abilities expressed extends, unavoidably, to the science of medicine on which they had pinned (and often continue to pin) so many of their hopes. As clinicians, we must give parents the space to be angry that medicine does not hold the answers they seek and recognize that some of that anger may actually be directed toward themselves.

No matter what they seem to think about their competence, clearly Brown and parents like him have become experts, if not in medicine, at least in their own child. They are certainly not failing at caregiving. Throughout the stories of frustration and disillusionment are moments of success. Walker Brown dissolves in hilarious laughter; Ted Hart finally understands how to tie his shoes; Ronan Rapp smiles; Sandy's son Jack takes one small step closer to toilet training. Next to the hopes they had once for their child, these steps may look insignificant. But in the day-to-day routine of caregiving they are no small thing. Parents must learn to celebrate the progress their child makes as he proceeds along his own line for development, never knowing if what they have done is enough, or if some other parent or approach or program would have been different. Despite the fact that clinicians also have no specific charts or guidelines for each child's unique path, and that success can be very difficult to recognize, we need to do our best to encourage them in celebrating these seemingly small things.

I believe that some extreme caregivers acquire knowledge of medical science as an integral part of their caregiving duties. But they do not measure their competence either by their ability to perform complex care or their scientific knowledge. They measure success as all parents do, by the accomplishments of their children.

It is clear that the task of extreme caregiving is difficult and requires a wide range of competencies. Despite the success of many parents at both accumulating medical knowledge and balancing a variety of duties, it is likely that there are parents who are unable to perform all or part of the task. Yet we assume routinely that every parent is not only willing, but also able, to take on this sort of care should their child require it. Given that even the most accomplished of these parents has doubts about their own competence, this assumption seems particularly questionable.

We cannot expect every parent to be good at every aspect of care. My father, with his selfish attitude toward intellectual disability and his privileged male upbringing, never changed a diaper, washed a bottle, or got up in the middle of the night for a feeding, though he worked diligently to earn the money that paid for them. He built the parallel bars with which my brother learned to walk, but he never held him and guided his footsteps through them. He never sat at the kitchen table wrestling with my brother's inability to grasp two plus two. But he recognized early that he needed to work to secure my brother's future. He fought for educational services, eventually overcoming his fear of public speaking to become president of the school Parent Teacher Association. His advocacy for the intellectually disabled was undeniable. It may be enough that he was competent in this one aspect of care, though my mother may never forgive him for ignoring my brother's other needs.

Certainly some parents become competent in medical knowledge as they search for explanations or solutions. This is admirable, but it is not the only form of competence that can be acquired. Nor can extensive knowledge of medicine become a mandatory requirement for either parent or family caregivers. Not all parents have the necessary resources, such as access to medical journals and the ability to understand them, access to a variety of professionals, or freedom to travel across the country for new programs or information. With the internet available to almost everyone, however, many parents are likely to attempt this search to the best of their abilities. It is possible that some parents perhaps are expecting too much from medicine and from themselves, and, lacking a realistic definition of success, they are unable to recognize their own competence. We do need to encourage this scientific competence by recognizing and promoting it when it happens.

It is unrealistic to expect families to provide round-the-clock care without a more extensive system of support. Spencer's care serves to illustrate the wide range of ability we expect from parents. Spencer's mother, who had not completed high school, and grandmother were doing well with much of his ICU-level nursing care. However, maximal support in their small community was not sufficient to provide all the care that, ideally, Spencer might need. The only possible next step, removing him from their care, seemed to me unreasonably intrusive and potentially damaging to all three of them. The lack of proper respite care, transportation, and education were Spencer's biggest problems, not maternal incompetence.

It seems likely that some children require too much care for a single family to provide, no matter how much financial and social support they receive. As Ian Brown states,

> There are political factions and even entire governments that . . . suggest that family is the only real solution to the problem of caring for the disabled. But families, like disabilities, are not uniform or consistent. They're anything but perfect . . . . As a result—this was my thinking—the nuclear family is no model for a system to care for the severely disabled. (2011, p 185)

He estimates that it would take six family members, living close together, to take care of Walker, if those people are to be permitted any other interests in their lives. This seems about right to me. Walker requires three eight-hour shifts per day, which would take at least five full-time people to cover nights and weekends. There are not enough people in the typical nuclear family to provide this degree of caregiving.

In addition, many extreme caregiving parents must fail in another goal of typical parenthood: launching the child into independent adulthood. The usual expectation is that parents are responsible for caring for their children until they grow to independence, at which point their job is more or less done. However, many children with special needs will never reach a point where they can live independently. Thus the caregiving task defined as parenting can never be completed or discontinued.

We have asked these parents to be competent at a task that is essentially impossible. Even if they can sustain the long hours and physical exertion, we cannot expect a parent to care for a dependent child forever. Eventually the child will become an adult who still requires care, and the parent will begin to need care themselves. I further review the problem of long-term care for people with intellectual disabilities in Chapter 8. For now, I will state that being unable at any point to care for the child at home cannot be labeled as failure. Greenfeld, Hart, and Brown, all of whom looked to placement outside their home for their sons in the teenage years, expressed their inability to continue home care in exactly that way. Their memoirs return repeatedly to the feelings of guilt over this perceived failure, adding an unnecessary and unfair burden to an already difficult task.

Perhaps the only way for extreme caregiving parents to discover their competence is in the small things; first steps taken at age seven, toilet training partially achieved at age twelve, or even figuring out why a fifteen-year-old, nonverbal child is upset. At times, success is measured merely by getting through the night. So these parents have no choice but to keep learning, working with their child, and completing the daily round of caregiving for as long as they can.

The goals of these parents are really the same as for every parent. They want their children to grow into unique individuals who can make their desires and personalities clear. They want to give them the best life possible and create for them a loving place in the world. They want to discover who their children are and who they might become. Promoting this form of growth is arguably the biggest task of parenting. Since the measurements applied in typical parenting provide no reliable guide to success, fulfilling this need is perhaps the most difficult aspect of extreme caregiving. We have seen that parents quest for medical knowledge as a way of understanding who their child is. In the next chapter, we look further into the moral work of maintaining and upholding an identity for a child who is nonverbal and cannot express his needs or his own life story without assistance.

CHAPTER 7 | Responsiveness

JOAN TRONTO (1993), in presenting her four phases of care, identified care-receiving as the fourth and most intimate phase of care. This is the final step in a cycle of care that begins with paying attention to needs, proceeds to taking a responsibility for meeting them, and leads to the performance of the hands-on tasks of caregiving. In this last phase, the caregiver calls forth a response from the care-receiver on both the quality and desirability of the care given. This phase makes it possible to bring new or different needs to the attention of the caregiver. Care can then be altered as desired, completing a feedback loop of caring. This both ensures that the care given is adequate and offers a safeguard against care that is unwanted or unnecessary.

Tronto assigned to the fourth phase, as its most important characteristic or necessary virtue, a quality she calls responsiveness. Responsiveness, she states, is similar to Kohlberg's earlier concept of reciprocity, which he considered to be an essential stage in moral development. According to Tronto, reciprocity is "the ability of [moral] reasoners to put themselves in the place of the other person in the dilemma" (1993, p. 67). In Kohlberg's theories of moral development, the advanced moral reasoner was thus able to understand that others may see the world differently and imagine how another might feel.

A more common understanding of reciprocity today is that it encompasses a mutual give-and-take process with another person. Responsiveness demands this sort of reciprocity but goes further. The responsive caregiver is asked not merely to empathically perceive the care-receiver's feelings but also to actually inquire about them. "Responsiveness suggests a different way to understand the needs of others rather than to put ourselves into their position. Instead, it suggests that we consider the other's position as that other expresses it" (Tronto, 1993, p. 136). The expressed needs revealed in turn create a new level of awareness, and the ability to return to the first phase of care with a deeper, and more accurate, level of attentiveness.

The crucial involvement of responsiveness in the caregiving cycle, suggests to me that caregiving as a moral act requires competence and responsiveness to exist side-by-side in the medical practitioner as two parallel virtues. Competence is needed in the daily work of medical care, which, at its bare minimum, deals with the maintenance of bodily health. But, as we have seen, parents desire more than that to consider themselves competent. They want to know their child's inner self and potential. Health care workers also desire to do more than callously administer medical science to bodies; they want to provide care for the whole patient. In order to do this, the patient must be seen as a person with a life narrative. For this person, encounters with the medical system are chapters in the story of their lives, and the providers of medicine are merely characters (Frank, 2002). The third phase requires the competent delivery of bodily care, but the fourth acknowledges the caregiver's involvement in the often changing, life narrative of the cared-for.

If responsiveness is absent, caregiving can be performed competently but only in a formulaic, impersonal sense. An example of competent caregiving that is lacking in responsiveness comes from the memoir *Bed Number Ten* by Sue Baier and Mary Zimmeth Schomaker (1989). In it, the narrator is temporarily rendered almost completely unresponsive by a rare paralytic illness called Guillain-Barré syndrome. She is intubated, tube fed, and unable to move anything except her eyelids. She is also uncomfortably warm. Her husband, during one of the short visits he is permitted, through a laborious, responsive process of "yes/no" blinks, manages to understand this and removes her blankets. For a short time, she is comfortable. However, after her husband leaves, her nurse, competently noticing the missing blankets and reciprocally assuming that she must be cold without them, promptly replaces them. The nurse has not taken the time to ask if this is needed. Perhaps she was unaware that her patient even had the ability to respond.

Martin Pistorius, in *Ghost Boy* (2013) provides an example of the opposite, an exquisite level of responsiveness. Martin has spent thirteen years conscious but unable to move voluntarily or communicate after being struck by a mysterious neurological disease at age twelve. He has been assessed as profoundly intellectually disabled, and most of his caregivers behave as though he cannot hear them. But a team of specialists in augmented communication, after careful observations of his eye movements and limited physical abilities, discover a way that he can answer questions. When they ask him if he would like to be able to make choices for himself, he isn't sure. He is not accustomed to making choices. He writes, "I know most people make thousands of decisions every day about what to eat and wear, where to go, and who to see, but I'm not sure I'll be able to make even one. It's like asking a child who has grown up in the desert to throw himself into the sea" (p. 29). Yet, one slow step at a time, he finds responsive people who listen to his needs and guide him to a life that includes a college degree, speaking engagements, and marriage.

Responsiveness as an action requires not merely an imagining of how the caregiver would feel in the care-receiver's position, but an actual inquiry into the care-receiver's needs. In practice, however, not everyone who needs care will be able to immediately and clearly express their exact needs. There are times when the moral caregiver is called upon to interpret the needs of a cared-for who will not, or cannot, respond. The caregiver must develop the skill of encouraging or eliciting a response to care from their charge. This is particularly true in situations of extreme dependency—young children, intellectual disability, severe illness, or dementia—where a coherent verbal response to care cannot be expected. In these cases, the caregiver might need to learn to interpret bodily needs and remain open to nonverbal cues from the cared-for. In order to complete the cycle of caring, the caregiver must be able to interpret the response to care from the care-receiver, in whatever manner it might come.

In extreme caregiving, verbal communication is often significantly delayed. Some children remain nonverbal, and their parents must rely entirely on physical reactions to bodily care. Often they are called upon to interpret their child's reactions for others. In the medical world, they must interpret signs and symptoms of illness, such as the severity or location of pain, and report them to providers. Their efforts become a bridge between the child and the outside world. The parent is given the responsibility of both providing for the child's needs and interpreting the response to that care.

It is in the act of interpreting and responding to the child's physical needs that many of the parent narrators discover who their child is, what his actions might mean, and where he might fit into the world. Parents look for cues from the child's reactions and interpret their meanings. Reactions to the environment, such as foods, music, or activities, become the basis for establishing likes and dislikes. The process of discovering their child's identity as a person thus occurs within the act of caregiving.

Responsiveness as a virtue becomes the basis for establishing individual personhood and creating a narrative for the child.

This chapter examines the ways in which parent extreme caregivers meet the challenge of responsiveness. I analyze the ways in which they look for a response and the ways in which they interpret both the child's needs and the child's personality despite limited verbal response. We shall see that the parents of older children who remain nonverbal acknowledge that their understanding is incomplete. Sometimes the mutual interactions involved in fulfilling the child's bodily needs are the only way the parent can establish a life story for the child. That narrative is the reason for their caregiving and gives meaning to both the child's life and their own.

Identity Formation and the Creation of a Life Story

To determine how stories are created in the context of caregiving, we must return briefly to the function of life narrative in the care of adults. Feminist philosopher Hilde Lindemann has proposed that families perform a narrative process, which she calls "holding in an identity" (2009). She maintains that families construct a narrative for each member, which becomes part of both the identity of the family member and the history of the family. Established over a lifetime, this narrative can help "hold the identity" of a person who is no longer able to participate actively in the telling of the story. In an essay on caring for patients (and family members) with dementia, Lindemann describes how a good caregiver can become a bridge to the past, a repository of memory of who the person used to be. She states that a family that is "holding well" will bestow and recognize humanity by remembering a life story already lived, thus "hold[ing] on to the demented person's identity for him or her" (2009, p. 416). This can be done by a family caregiver, or by a responsive outside caregiver to whom some of the stories have been passed. The knowledge of a person's life, who they are or who they were, will, of course, add respect and understanding to the caregivers' ability to respond.

Adults who encounter serious illness already have a series of past experiences from which the caregiver can derive understanding of their evolving life story. Narrative ethicists Arthur Frank (1995, 1997) and Howard Brody (1997, 2003) both support the idea that situating a patient within a life narrative can provide a framework for improved care. They suggest that a physician or caregiver might participate in the narrative of illness by becoming a witness to the suffering written on the body of the ill patient.

Frank recommends that clinicians, by listening to a patient's life story, can help write a new story that incorporates the changes brought about by the unexpected presence of illness. Both of these frameworks essentially involve upholding or maintaining an identity for a person who has stepped out of their expected life story and into a new narrative composed of illness.

Knowing about the life narrative of the cared-for helps the caregiver provide better care. By accurately understanding the way in which a patient's needs fit into his or her life, the caregiver is better able to both elicit and understand that patient's response to care. If the caregiver knows about the life of the cared-for, then the caregiver can better interpret their response, as well, particularly if the person who requires care is verbally compromised.

An adult care-receiver with dementia (or an illness that has compromised their mental capacity) has previously been the author and protagonist of their own story. The virtuous caregiver must (merely) discover and understand it. A responsive caregiver for an adult can, in most situations, elicit a response to care and/or relate to a story already at least partly told. But this does not seem to be the case for infants and small children for whom there is, as yet, not much of a life story to act on.

Looking more closely, however, the life story of even a newborn infant is already surprisingly complex. Most obviously, infants hold the promise of a vast and varied future, an individual story that is just beginning. They also are already placed into the ongoing story of their family. Lindemann (2009) has pointed out that family holding often begins before a child is born, with a family making a place for the new child-to-be. The infant is added to an already existing story wherein the identities of parents, siblings, relatives, and neighbors are held. The infant joins a narrative that is constantly developing, and sends that story on a new trajectory which includes the potential within that newborn life.

All parents, by expecting and preparing for their child's future, are bringing forth and in many ways creating their child as a unique human being. As the first narrator of their child's life, the parent has an enormous responsibility, and must become deeply involved in the child's story. At first the story of the child's life is comprised largely of her place in the family and that family's expectations for her future.

As the infant begins to interact with the family, her unique story slowly grows. The care that the new infant receives, along with her responses to it, becomes part of the family story (Lindemann, 2014). As they interact through the daily routine of caregiving, parent and child discover each other. A baby might spit out certain foods, or calm only when held in a certain way, or gaze at a bright object. Any of these actions can be interpreted by the family as early evidence of personality traits. As the child grows and develops the ability to make her preferences clearer, her story becomes more individualized. Once she can express her desires verbally, the child can begin to tell her own story, which continues to be entwined with the family's story and forms a part of the identity of both.

Once the child becomes verbal, she can begin to question the identity and narrative that has been laid out for her. A family that is "holding well" will have allowed freedom for the child to tell her own story and establish her own identity. Philosopher Joel Feinberg has called this the "right to an open future," saying that children should have as many options as possible available when they finally attain the ability to autonomously choose between them (Feinberg, 1980). A careful parent must remain open to alternative futures and avoid placing restrictive expectations on their child. A careful parent will also guard the child's unique narrative, along with guarding the child's future, so that the story that eventually emerges is the child's own authentic story.

The recognition of a disability or the diagnosis of an illness interrupts those emerging expectations, altering the story of both child and family. It should not be surprising that families experience a time of disorientation and grieving as they come to terms with the unexpectedly different narrative.

Families not only have to learn to cope with different expectations, but they must also depend for a longer time on the interpretations gained from meeting bodily needs. In many of the children requiring extreme caregiving, the emergence of the child's unique story is delayed along with the child's development. Disability or illness also can delay the arrival of the time when the child can be her own spokesperson in her emerging story. In some, there is never a coherent or reliable response. This is clearly of paramount importance to many of the authors of extreme caregiving narratives, who, as we have seen, struggle to understand their child's identity and discover their unique story.

Emily Rapp (2013), whose son Ronan had Tay-Sachs, a fatal neurodegenerative disease, writes in her memoir that she considered finding her son's story one of her main tasks in caring for him. The disease causes progressive neurological destruction, so Ronan barely reached a developmental level of six months before regressing into unresponsiveness. She writes, "My other task beyond physical care, I began to realize, was to find Ronan's quiet, gap-ridden myth, his idiosyncratic narrative—to interpret it, share it, and learn from it" (p. 48). In the act of writing her memoir, she tries to make sense of his limited world, looking to poetry, myth, and philosophy, to try to discover Ronan's place in the world and understand his experience of life.

She knows that the story she tells for him will be the only one he will ever have. She continues:

> What if Ronan "described" his experiences to me? Would a touch be feathery? No, he had no concept of a feather. Words and descriptions were meaningless abstractions. He was simply going forward every moment and leaving everything behind. No analysis, no memory, no stress, no desire. He let everything pass; he let it all get lost. In that gap where he existed there was no map for his meaning. *But there would be*, I thought. If Ronan needed a myth, I would write one. If the only way to stop being divided from him, if the only way to dwell in his space, even for a moment, which I ardently, desperately wanted to do, was to stare into that silent world and make it speak, then I had work to do. (pp. 48–49)

In order to be responsive to her son's story, Rapp became the only coherent narrator of Ronan's life. In doing this, she had to both ask what Ronan needed and interpret his silent answer. It is moral work to reach outside oneself and give voice to someone who is voiceless.

Very few parents are called upon to do what Rapp did for her son Ronan; to find, with almost no evidence, that "quiet, gap-ridden myth, his idiosyncratic narrative" (p. 48). Fortunately, most parents enjoy an increasing level of interaction rather than a child's progressive neurological diminishment. Most parents also have considerably more time in which to frame their child's life narrative. However, the parent extreme caregiver is often called upon to both interpret and meet the needs of a child whose responses are minimal or unreliable. The parent must maintain both parts of the responsiveness cycle, both query and answer, for an extended period of time. And we shall see that guarding the distant, uncertain future is ultimately an act of infinite patience and creativity. It is also an act which requires moral judgment.

The Hazards of Responsiveness

Portia Iversen's son Dov was diagnosed with autism shortly after his twelve-month check-up. By age nine, he had regressed in some developmental milestones and was still unable to speak or communicate in any way. So when she heard about Tito, a boy with a similar degree of autism, but who was able to write poetry on the internet, she was both intrigued and seized by an impossible hope. She invited Tito and his mother Soma from their home in India to Los Angeles and wrote about the experience in a 2006 book called *Strange Son: Two Mothers, Two Sons, and the Quest to Unlock the Hidden World of Autism.*

Iversen had already founded Cure Autism Now (CAN), an advocacy group dedicated to bringing together neuroscientists and funding research in autism. It was through this group that Iversen funded Tito and Soma's trip from India, initially as a keynote speaker at a CAN Innovative Technology for Autism conference. In front of an audience, Tito immediately displayed signs of autism, "rocking and flapping ... so much that it looked like he might levitate at any moment" (2006, p. 47). But then, at his mother's command, he began tapping out letters on a hastily made alphabet board. Iversen reports, "'*Hello*' was all Tito had to tap out before the audience was on their feet in thunderous applause" (p. 48). He went on to answer questions, mostly about what it was like to have autism, from the audience and later in individual sessions. He communicated by pointing at a letter board, handwriting with a pencil, or typing on a keyboard, always with his mother by his side.

Iversen was convinced that Tito held a key, not only to communicating with her own son, but also to understanding and, therefore, curing autism. In an attempt to "figure out autism through Tito" (p. 53), she scheduled appointments with scientists across the country to study Tito. It did not go well. Iversen describes bouts of uncontrollable and sometimes destructive behavior, often interfering with the testing. She also describes constant repetitive behaviors such as flapping, rocking, grinding his teeth, or pacing— activities associated with autism and commonly called self-stimulation, or "stimming." Tito could not sit still or follow instructions. He could not perform self care. He ate by messily stuffing food into his mouth. He often engaged in energetic and sometimes alarming stimming between words, requiring his mother to direct his attention back to whichever communication method he had been using.

As the testing proceeded, it became increasingly obvious that Tito's mother was an integral part of the process of communication. Soma reported to Iversen the painstaking and prolonged process by which she had trained Tito to, first, point at letters, then progress to forming them on paper or typing them. She also recognized that Tito was not able to process information from the world around him, and so she provided for him "a continuous narrative in which she explained everything in their world"

(p. 87). She read books to him also, stopping after one or two sentences to make sure he had heard and understood them. She prodded him continuously, shouting "C'mon!" to focus his attention. Through this method, Tito learned math, literature, science, and poetry.

To teach him, Soma needed to be constantly at his side and constantly aware of his world. Soma reported to Iversen that she had to observe the pattern of Tito's stimming and learn to outpace and override it. "You had to look at how the child stims, she said, observe the pace of it. And you had to go faster. The autistic child is constantly distracted, so *you* have to be the biggest destracter of all. 'You have to *become* the stim!' Soma declared" (p. 325). His mother found a way to reach Tito by interpreting and overcoming the noise in his brain, and helping him to keep the channels open. Iversen says, "Soma had to conduct Tito's arousal activity like an orchestra, to keep it in a range where he could attend to the information she was presenting long enough to encode it" (p. 338).

On the surface this seems to be the ultimate in responsiveness. Soma not only attended to Tito's physical needs—bathing him, and dressing him, and brushing his teeth—but she also dedicated her life to understanding him and helping him be understood. By observing the world for him and narrating it to him at a pace that meshed with his disordered senses, she was the first audience for his thoughts and provided the first response to them. Through her, Tito found a voice.

There was, however, an obvious problem with this system. Tito was unable to perform without his mother's presence. He could not read without her at his side, prodding him to keep going. He could not follow any information that was read or said to him by others. He only rarely wrote or typed without her by his side.

A technique similar to Soma's, called facilitated communication, gained popularity in the late 1980s but had already fallen out of favor by the time Tito and his mother came to the United States. The technique was carried out by a facilitator, who steadied the arm or hand of a person with limited muscle control, so that they could communicate by pointing to pictures or letters on a board. Researchers were unable to replicate the communication independently, however, and psychologists theorized that many facilitators were subconsciously moving the patient's hand for them. The potential for abuse of this method is high, as facilitators can fabricate conversations and possibly entire personalities. Recently, in 2015, a facilitator was convicted of sexual assault, after convincing herself that she and a young man she was helping were in love (Engber, 2015).

I will not belabor the possibility that Tito's abilities were at least partially faked, or, as one scientist Iversen interviewed put it, "An elaborate smoke and mirrors" (2006, p. 62). If Tito's mother was fabricating his attempts at communication, the ethical implications are clear. Tito becomes the subject of an abusive relationship, passively participating in a sort of magic act performed on him by his mother. However, Tito's mother merely needed to be present for him to communicate; she did not need to interact with Tito physically. The length and depth of conversations carried on with Tito and observed by Iversen, make such a performance nearly impossible. I will assume that Soma really had, with great effort and responsiveness, opened up a narrow channel through which her son's genius but autistic mind, could speak. Even then, there are still some disturbing ethical questions raised by this method of communication.

The first question is the level of devotion required from Soma. She invested her life in Tito's needs—seemingly subsumed her own needs to enable Tito's communication. She left behind a husband and family who could not deal with Tito's needs and behavior in order to be constantly by his side. It seems unfair to ask her to do this, but it is difficult to criticize responsiveness that takes over the life of a parent, particularly when that parent is taking care of a child who likely will not thrive in any other environment. Yet Soma had chosen to invest her life in such a way and cannot really be judged for doing so.

My biggest concern, however, is for Tito. At the time the book was written, he was a seemingly highly intelligent fourteen-year-old boy trapped in a brain that could neither attend to his environment nor communicate with the world, unless his mother was present. As Iversen explains,

> Tito himself was incapable of initiating anything. I had never seen Tito ask for his alphabet board or pad of paper, or even reach for them when they were nearby. Instead, he would sit and listen, rocking and flapping feverishly until Soma thought to hand him a blank pad of paper or his alphabet board. Only then would he have the chance to blurt out his thoughts on paper. He was totally at the mercy of Soma to realize that he might have something to say and to help him do so. (pp. 118–119)

The limitation inherent in this process is evident. Tito was dependent on his mother's responsiveness to connect him to the world. In order to say anything, he needed his mother to prod him.

By being dependent on Soma to keep the channels to the outside world open, Tito was also dependent on her to choose the information that passed through those channels. Since Tito was unable to process the chaotic information that came through his senses, he relied on his mother's descriptions. She chose what Tito saw and heard by describing things for him. She chose the books he read and asked questions to focus him on the information she thought was important.

If Soma did not want Tito to know about something, she merely did not mention it to him. Presumably if she did not want him to talk about something, she could simply withdraw her support. She admits, for example, that she never talked about anything personal with Tito. There were times that Soma inexplicably refused to cooperate with a conversation or testing for Tito, raising the suspicion that territory that she did not want explored had been broached. Iversen recognized the difficulty of having only a single line to the outside world. "Imagine: Your mind thinks, creates ideas and thoughts," she writes, "You forge a tiny pathway to the outer world to express them, but you need someone else to initiate the use of this pathway. And when the person does initiate for you, they must constantly prompt you along and keep you in your chair long enough to write out what is in your mind" (pp. 178–179). Iversen recognized the essential loneliness of being so isolated, adding, "If Soma was the only person Tito could communicate with and she never talked about anything personal Tito must be even more lonely and isolated than I had imagined" (p. 124). Iversen was aware of how difficult this must be for Tito, to need someone else to provide access to the world.

However Iversen never acknowledged the awesome power that Soma wielded over her son. Soma controlled everything that went into and out of her son's mind. He had never been able to explore the world for himself, perhaps to follow a direction that interested him and not his mother. He had never been able to express a thought in private from his mother. Even if his mother was holding him well and guarding an open future for him, to the best of her ability, Tito's every word was still subject to his mother's scrutiny and interpretation. He will never be able to go out into the world to explore the future without parental influence and bias. His identity must remain buried in hers.

And there is some evidence that Soma was not using her power in an entirely altruistic manner. Tito's mother could control him, through directing his attention, and seemed to have no intention of letting anyone else into their private world. She actively resisted any attempt to communicate with Tito in her absence. She was also uninterested in teaching anyone else her techniques, though she did begin to teach Iversen's son Dov. But just as Dov was beginning to learn to talk using a letter board, Soma abruptly moved to another state. Iversen regretted the loss of a teacher but never questioned her motives.[1]

Tito at least had some ability to determine his own self. It is likely that his development as a unique person will continue despite the necessity of his mother's involvement. Judging from the enormous amounts of his work included in *Strange Son*, Tito emerged as a literate, thoughtful individual. He wrote poetry that expressed the feelings and emotions he could not express verbally, and told his own very unique story. Iversen repeatedly states that his main desire was for his writing to be published, to have his voice be heard, but she does not speculate about the difficulties that might arise for Tito in the future, if there is only one person who is able to hold the pathway open for him.

Not all who require the sort of care that Tito needs will find a way to express themselves so eloquently. There are children, including other children with autism, such as Noah Greenfeld, who never find a pathway through which they can communicate. There are children like Walker Brown and Savannah, who can communicate only through gestures and signs. Others, like my brother, learn words slowly and with great difficulty, and can express themselves only in the most basic of words. All of these children are dependent on their caregivers to remain open and responsive, to interpret fairly their actions and desires, and to create a story that is a true reflection of the child's authentic self, no matter how hidden it might be.

It is an immense responsibility, and one that ties parent to child in an inextricable, often permanent bond. One mother, whose son Wolf has multiple disabilities due to a syndrome called Velocardiofacial syndrome (VCFS), writes, "I am closer to Wolf than I was to my own mother, closer to Wolf than I ever was to my husband or my best friend. Closer than I am to [my daughter]. Wolf and I are actually a part of each other. This is forever, I realize now. He is not going to outgrow me. He needs me to complete his thoughts" (Carver, 2007, pp. 34–35). The bond, formed out

---

[1] Soma moved to Texas, where she now runs an organization called HALO: Helping Autism through Learning and Outreach via which she teaches the method she used to reach Tito, now called "rapid prompting method" or RPM. On the website, she offers personal educational evaluations and teaching, as well as seminars, which are scheduled exclusively through inquiries on the website. About *Strange Son*, the site says, "We generally appreciate those who work towards autism efforts. However, Soma and HALO's position differs from the author, title and book, which we do not endorse" (halo-soma.org, retrieved April 10, 2016). The site sells books by both Tito and Soma, but is not up to date. Tito Mukhopadhyay's most recent book, *Plankton Dreams: What I Learned in Special-Ed*, published in 2015, is not listed, but is available on line from Open Humanities Press.

of responsiveness to the day-to-day meeting of needs, can be perilous for both caregiver and cared-for, as both can be lost in, but also enriched by, their shared identity.

Responsiveness seems to me to be a virtue the exercise of which is of enormous moral consequence. Extreme caregiving becomes a task that must be conducted with wisdom and patience. Parents seeking to understand who their child is, and to help their child thrive to their maximum potential, must take care not to impose their hopes and expectations on a child who becomes entwined with them and may never be able to contradict them.

The Child Is Not the Disease

One of the first places many parents look for knowledge of the child's identity is in the child's body. The first steps in family identity formation might come from observations of physical characteristics, such as gender, but the earliest relationship is created from the interactions necessary for caregiving. The identity that a family will hold for a child emerges from physical holding. Feeding, bathing, and even diaper changes become a way of getting to know each other. Many family interactions with an infant begin within the context of caregiving and the newborn infant's response to that care.

Following the discovery, or even the suspicion of a medical problem, parents are often called upon to alter care in a variety of ways. Even a minor feeding difficulty might result in multiple medical visits and the incorporation of new nursing techniques. If the infant requires specialized medical care at home, the parents' first foray into the acquisition of medical knowledge might center on learning to provide home treatments or respond to medical crises. The child's survival may depend on incorporation of this new knowledge into the way the family cares for the child. The medical procedures, and the labels that come with them, become part of the identities of both infant and family.

As we saw in Chapter 6, some parents search for further medical knowledge and become unacknowledged experts in the diagnosis and treatment of their children's medical problems. They do not abandon this activity even if it becomes clear there is no definitive cure or treatment available. The search often continues despite a resulting disillusionment with medicine and becomes instead a way of understanding the child outside the realm of diagnosis. This is one way to establish and hold an identity for the child within the family.

The presence of an illness or disability will unavoidably alter the evolving story of the child's life. We have seen that this can occur quite early in the child's story, sometimes before birth, if there is a prenatal diagnosis of a genetic syndrome. Understanding the disease is a way to determine how the child's life story, both present and future, has been altered from expectations. Learning as much as possible about the medical consequences of a disability allows the creation of a new story and the reworking of possible futures. It is also a way for the family to come to terms with the changes in their own lives that will occur from becoming caregivers for a child with special needs.

For many children with special needs, it is inevitable that their illness or disability becomes some part of the definition of who they are. Its presence has unavoidably rewritten the narrative of their lives. I once asked the mother of a child with Cornelia DeLange syndrome (CDLS), if she ever wished that her son had been born without all of the problems that syndrome brought him. Samuel was developmentally delayed, still a toddler at age nine years, and had a variety of medical problems that made his long-term life expectancy uncertain. Her answer surprised me. She said that she could have no regrets, because Samuel has CDLS, and a child without CDLS would be a different child. The child that she has, and loves, is Samuel. Samuel's story is inextricable from CDLS; to have a different body would mean being a different child.

Michael Berube, scholar and father of Jamie, who has Down syndrome, writes, "I do not waste my time . . . thinking about what Jamie would be like if he did not have Down syndrome; if he did not have Down syndrome, he would not be Jamie. We love him for the person he is, and do not worry about the person he might have been if he were an entirely different person" (2016, p. 48). Again, the child's disability and the child's identity are inseparable, though it is important to remember that Down syndrome is only part of Jamie's identity: he defines it, it does not define him. Samuel also is a child with a disabling syndrome, but though it must be a part of who he is, CDLS is not his entire identity.

Emily Rapp, the author of a memoir about her son's brief life with Tay-Sachs disease, agrees, though she is somewhat ambivalent. Remembering the experience of an ordinary day with Ronan, she says, "I rolled through the grocery store with my floppy, beautiful boy and some days I wouldn't have had it any other way because to wish otherwise would be to wish for another baby, which I did not." Given the fact of his illness and impending death, however, she continues, "On other days I railed against this fact and wished I could . . . do the impossible" (2013,

p. 184). She wishes for the ability to cure him, yet she knows that this is impossible, both because there is no cure and because a different body would have made him a different child.

Not all parents are as accepting of the child's disabilities as part of their true selves, however. Ian Brown, whose son Walker has a rare genetic syndrome called CFC, reports that his wife Johanna does not think of Walker's CFC as being a part of him.

> "I hear parents of other handicapped kids saying all the time, 'I wouldn't change my child,'" Johanna said one night as we were lying in bed, talking as we fell asleep. "They say, 'I wouldn't trade him for anything.' But I would. I would trade Walker, if I could push a button, for the most ordinary kid who got C's in school. I would trade him in an instant. I wouldn't trade him for my sake, for our sake. But I would trade for his sake. I think Walker has a very, very hard life." (2011, p. 80)

Johanna is also not interested in meeting other children with CFC, an experience which for her husband is part of understanding Walker. She wants to see Walker only as himself and is afraid that knowledge of others like him will make her start seeing him as "a kid with a syndrome" (p. 113). But for Brown, the experience of meeting other children with CFC is monumental. He says, "Even the briefest meeting with another CFC child felt like the discovery of a new element" (p. 120). But, like Samuel, Jamie, and Ronan, none of the children with CFC can entirely escape the stories defined for them by their bodies, though, of course, the story witnessed in their bodies cannot be their whole story.

Parents of typical children also look for information to help them understand their child, particularly guidance regarding child development, though for the parents of children with special needs, this search is more medicalized and often more intense. Jennifer Graf Groneberg, the mother of an infant with Down syndrome (DS), read a pile of books on development in children with DS. But she compares this to reading standard books on child development after the birth of her first child. She writes, "My feelings are familiar, and my motives are similar. I want to feel like I understand Avery so that I can support him, and be a good mother to him, as he grows. I want to figure out my son (Groneberg, 2008, p. 187). In order to for Avery to thrive with DS, his mother must learn all she can about the syndrome. This knowledge will help her understand and hold his identity, just as reading about typical development helped her guide her first child.

Parents whose children remain nonverbal past the toddler years often begin to concentrate their studies on language acquisition. They look both for ways to encourage communication and ways to interpret the clues they do receive. For Greenfeld (1970), Hart (1989), and Iversen (2006), whose sons with autism were nonverbal, the quest for medical knowledge became a quest for a connection with their sons. Greenfeld traveled widely in search of therapies to reach his son. Hart also pursued medical treatments that would break through the communication barrier, with the goal of understanding his son as an individual. Iversen is perhaps unique in her ability to found an organization to fund autism research, but her ultimate goal was to be able to talk to her nonverbal son. For all three, understanding autism became a literal attempt to understand their child, the only way to discover who their child was.

Parents seeking to know their child rarely find the child's identity in the medical diagnosis, however. At some point, many parents learn instead to fight this medical identity, to avoid seeing their child as a disease. Some develop an understandable resentment toward the clinical aspects of medicine and those practitioners who see only the disability and not the child. I am reminded of a phrase frequently used during my pediatric training: "The child is not the disease." This is a reminder aimed at professional caregivers to pay attention to more than the child's medical chart, to see the child as a whole person beyond the illness or disability, and to consider the needs of the child situated within a family.

Ian Brown (2011) studies the genetics of CFC in detail and comes to resent the picture of his son Walker as merely a genetic defect. He realizes that Walker's body is not his whole story. When describing Walker's body, as he does near the beginning of *The Boy in the Moon*, it is evident that Brown knows this. He describes his son's unusual body in poetic terms: "His shoulder blades and the bones of his back are oddly soft, plastic, bendable, as if covered by some miracle upholstery. The skin of his arms and thighs feels almost manufactured too, too much matte and not enough flow, the cells rampaging, overbuilding, one of the more direct results of the genetic miscues that made him this way" (p. 12). Despite the use of mechanical and clinical words, something individual and beautiful shines through. He calls Walker "my sweet, sweet, lost and broken boy" (p. 7).

Walker is more than his disease, more even than his genetic makeup, and those medical professionals whose job it is to elucidate Walker's problems are often unable to hear his whole story. In this quote from *The Boy in the Moon*, Brown describes both the realization that Walker is not his syndrome and the disconnect that often occurs between parents and professionals who fail to recognize the difference. It also is a testimony to the sorrow that results from the "broken" body that sets Walker apart from other children. Brown writes,

> [T]o a laboratory geneticist who studied CFC as a genetic disorder, the syndrome was always *only* that: a disorder, an unfixable spelling mistake in the grammar of humanness. I understood that stance, and also hated it. Seeing Walker only as a genetic disorder was a guaranteed way for me to remember that there is such a thing as genetic *order*, that for each Walker, there are millions of genetically complete children. In a genetics lab, Walker would always be a deleterious effect of nature and evolution, and little more. (2011, p.177)

To Brown, Walker must be more than the genetic mutation that produced his syndrome. Brown must become the one who recognizes the "more" that Walker is, and the one on whom the burden of discovering what that "more" might be falls. He must find and nurture Walker's true self and his full story.

Crafting a Narrative for a Nonverbal Child

I have said that the formation of a child's identity begins in infancy, as parents interpret and respond to bodily needs. As they perform routine caregiving, parents form their first ideas about the child's personality and begin to craft a life story for him. But they really have very little information on which to base their narrative. Even when caring for typical infants, as most parents could attest, it is not always easy to interpret physical needs.

One of the most frustrating medial problems in the neonate, for parent and pediatrician alike, is colic. This is marked by inconsolable and inexplicable crying, and it occurs in infants from age two weeks to about four months. The parent, of course, has a mental list of things that might cause a baby to cry so much: hunger, cold, dirty diapers, pain, heat, constipation. One by one, those possibilities are checked, and remedied if possible, yet the baby's crying continues. The parent cannot help but imagine some horrible pain, with terrible consequences if its source is overlooked. The pediatrician also has a long mental list of possibilities, most of which can be discarded because of a lack of corroborating symptoms or lab abnormalities. There are formulas to try and advice to be given, but the pediatrician knows no more than the parent. There is no evidence, except for the crying, that something is wrong. The baby can't tell anyone what, if anything, hurts.

Infants "outgrow" this problem eventually, of course. And sooner or later, when something does hurt, children become able to at least point to the "owie." But many children with special needs are unable to reliably report on their needs until much later, if at all. This leaves the extreme caregiver in much the same situation as the parent of a colicky infant; if the child seems distressed, they often have to guess not just about what the problem might be but also whether there is actually a problem.

Two nurses who studied the mothers of children with severe chronic illness or disabilities, McKeever and Miller, noted that mothers have a remarkable ability to interpret their child's needs and that a strong bond forms between maternal caregiver and the child cared for at home. They do not have statistics for how often mothers are correct about their child's needs, but they do provide several narratives from parents whose concerns were ignored, some resulting in inadequate care. They state that the mothers learned to "accurately determine, respond to, and compensate for children's physical needs and multiple vulnerabilities," and, as a result, "their need for vigilant attention to subtle physiological, behavioural and emotional cues led to extremely close relationships. Mothers 'knew' the children in a way few others did and were uniquely attuned to them" (McKeever & Miller, 2004, p. 1182). I also have found that the parents of children with special health care needs are uniquely attuned to their child's physical needs. If, for example, a mother of a child with multiple medical problems says that she thinks her child is becoming very sick and should be in the hospital, I have found it best to hospitalize that child because she is very likely right. The parents are not always correct, of course, but often enough.

But the need for responsiveness extends to more than maintenance of physical needs, no matter how difficult they are to establish. The interpretation of emotional needs, particularly those that build a story of the child's identity, is even more difficult. Parents might ascribe various personality traits to a colicky baby, for example. Perhaps it is evidence that the child is finicky, or sickly, or uncooperative. Or, if the crying is particularly fierce, parents might claim that the child is a "fighter."

During many visits with my friend Annette, our conversation was frequently interrupted by her daughter Savannah's attempts to communicate. Savannah had CFC, the same syndrome as Walker Brown. At age nineteen, Savvy had no words, but she did use some sign language. Over the years,

Annette and Savvy had invented a different sign for each of the many people in her life; each family member, caregiver, therapist, and teacher was assigned a specific area of the body to which Savvy pointed. Savvy often asked about these people by pointing to the person's individual body part. At each gesture, her mother said the person's name, and gave an often detailed report about where they might be and what they might be doing at the moment. Savannah sometimes laughed, or clapped, or cried, but more often she just immediately pointed somewhere else. Her mother's days were filled with responding to a ceaseless, and to me seemingly random, pointing. Annette took this as evidence that Savvy was very loving and cared deeply for all the people she knew. I was often convinced that the real point for Savvy was to draw her mother's attention back to her and away from distractions. Both of us could be wrong.

And yet, through a combination of these minimal signs and an intimate knowledge of her daughter's schedule and interests, I have also seen Annette understand some fairly complex messages. One message, translated with some difficulty, was that one of Savvy's favorite teachers had driven her home from school that day, honked her horn once in the driveway, and was going to do both things again tomorrow. This seemed to me to be a bit of a stretch for a sequence of pointing and crying. But Savvy's obvious delight made it clear that Annette's interpretation was correct. She had to repeat all the parts of the message at least ten times, each time accompanied by laughter and clapping.

Looking for the unique self of the noncommunicative or unreliably communicative child is not easy. Parents may be searching diligently and honestly to discover who their child is, but there are very few clues to go on. This is the source of the title of Ian Brown's book, the *Boy in the Moon*. Walker is able to give Brown very few clues about himself. "Sometimes," Brown writes, "watching Walker is like looking at the moon: you see the face of the man in the moon, yet you know there's actually no man there" (2011, p. 3). Despite all of Brown's efforts and reasoning, Walker remains as inscrutable as the man in the moon.

The *Boy in the Moon* is full of attempts to interpret and understand Walker's unusual behaviors, but Brown is aware of the limitations of his knowledge. For example, Walker likes to play with plastic bags full of pop can tabs or, rather, this specific "toy" focuses Walker's attention repeatedly. Brown fills several paragraphs with musings as to what Walker might be enjoying about the sensation of kneading a bag of pop can tabs, if indeed he is enjoying it. The section becomes a flight of fantasy as to what this means to his son, or what anything might mean to his son. He concludes, "Or maybe I am reaching. He gives me no choice but to reach this way. He and I invent our world together every moment I am with him" (p. 15).

At age three Walker begins hurting himself, hitting himself and banging his head hard enough to cause injury. The source of this self-injurious behavior is a mystery that requires an urgent answer. However Brown never finds one.

> Sometimes Walker was in agony as he smacked himself and screamed with pain. At other times he seemed to do it more expressively, as a way to clear his head, or to let us know he would be saying something if he could talk. Sometimes—and this was unbearably sad—he laughed immediately afterwards. He couldn't tell us anything, and we had to imagine everything. (p. 77)

Walker sometimes laughs in response to self-injury, when he must be in pain. Yet at other times, he laughs, delighting his father, who is pleased by this evidence that his hard-to-read son is happy. Brown has no choice but to respond to the outward signs of his son's feelings since he has so little access to the feelings themselves. If Brown is to be a responsive caregiver, caring for his son's story as well as his body, he must construct a narrative from the few facts he is given, inconsistent though they may be.

Feminist philosopher Eva Kittay is the mother of a daughter with profound intellectual disabilities, Sesha. In an essay about her daughter, Kittay reports that Sesha "has no measurable IQ" and that there are many "capacities she will not develop at all" (1999, p. 151). Yet to Kittay, and also to Peggy, her paid caregiver for over two decades, Sesha is a unique individual full of boundless joy and love and a certain amount of stubbornness. Sesha does not talk, or walk, or even eat, yet in a later paper, Kittay describes her as having "her own personality, her own mature beauty" and as becoming "increasingly mature emotionally" (2011, p. 614). Kittay admits that her understanding of her daughter is incomplete, but so is our understanding of all others, even those who can communicate fully. She writes:

> I have come to grow increasingly more humble in what I think I know about my daughter . . . The quality of containment, of mystery that we each present to each other, regardless of ability, is increasingly clear to me. We always see each other through a glass darkly, but when viewing a child with cognitive disabilities, the glass is darker still. (2011, p. 614)

Kittay and Peggy, while likely Sesha's best and only interpreters, have very little information to work with. Their responsiveness in caregiving must include a large amount of uncertainty.

Kittay describes a happy day for Sesha, in which she gives her caregiver, Peggy, a kiss. Kittay describes Sesha's kisses as "legendary" and "distinctive," with "mouth open, top teeth lightly (and sometimes not so lightly) pressing on your cheek, her breath full of excitement and happiness, her arms around your neck (if you're lucky; if not, arms up, hands on hair, which caveman-like, she uses to pull your face to her mouth)" (1999, pp. 150–151). This could describe other things, as Sesha tangles her fingers in someone's hair and pulls them into her bared teeth, but Kittay says it is a kiss. Kittay and apparently also Peggy interpret this as an expression of Sesha's boundless love and joy. They are probably right.

Noah Greenfeld, at age three, has a perhaps similar kiss, described by Greenfeld. His wife, Foumi, "claims that [Noah] sometimes comes over to her and presses his lips against hers." Greenfeld continues, "And at times he does the same thing to me. But I'm convinced he's considering more a bite than a kiss on those occasions—and sometimes I have the tooth nibble marks to prove it" (1970, p. 183). Noah's two primary caregivers, witnessing the same action, disagree on its meaning. There is no way to determine who is correct.

Much of the interpretation of clues centers on the child's happiness. Angie Lydicksen, mother of Luke, another child with CFC, who was interviewed by Ian Brown, told him:

> "I think Luke, for the most part, he's happy," Angie said. "When he does cry, he usually cries for a reason. I think his quality of life is good, for the most part—I think he's happy in his own little world. And for the most part I'm happy that he's happy. Sometimes it breaks your heart, because he's stuck in his own little world. But sometimes I wonder if it's not better there. Sometimes—because he goes to bed with a smile and wakes up with a smile—I like to think he's happy all the time. I like to think he is." (2011, p. 155)

She thinks he is happy. But she does not know, and will never know, for sure. So she monitors his body for signs of pain or illness, and monitors his moods as best she can, and hopes that he is happy when nothing seems to be wrong.

Emily Rapp, who knows that her son is regressing into a vegetative state and death from Tay-Sachs disease, also wonders about his happiness, but is less convinced.

> Was Ronan unhappy? No. He had no label for that.
> Are we any happier when we know (or think we know) the difference between unhappy and happy? I doubt it. Life is really lived within those parentheticals, in what we don't know or expect, in what has already disappeared, in what is already gone. When Ronan's sensory faculties disappeared, did that mean that his narrative went with it, or did he simply exist in that gap, a place we could not access without relinquishing the desire to understand its parameters, to make sense of it? (2013, p. 46)

She finds his story by living in the brief moments of joy and connectedness she has with him, but, simultaneously, she is unable to forget the dismal future ahead. Ronan's story is in those moments of happiness, described in glorious detail. His narrative, while informed by death, is not a story about dying. The inevitable death looms, but his mother does not describe his death in her book.

Some of the parent narrators we have been examining doubt their own abilities as parents and caregivers because they cannot fully understand their nonverbal child. Hart, whose son Ted has autism, admits that sometimes he and his wife could not "trust our own judgment when it came to making decisions about Ted's future.... We had lost a sense of proportion and couldn't gauge whether our efforts were enough, too much, or too little" (1989, p. 183). And Brown admits, "I often wondered if we were imagining Walker's progress, inventing the connections we thought he was making" (2011, p. 38). He also has no way to confirm that his efforts are sufficient and suspects that any progress Walker makes is imaginary.

The uncertainty extends to wondering, not only what Walker might say, if he could, but also whether he is aware of the story his father is creating for him. Brown writes,

> To hear him speak his own name? . . . To hear him say, *Ma, I love you?* My heart is banging at the thought. *Fuck you, Dada!* would be the Gettysburg Address . . . . I don't need to Walker to say *I love you* to know he does. But if he spoke a word, it would be proof that he had something to say and that he wanted to say it, that there was a point to his saying it. (pp. 124—125)

He knows Walker's limitations; Walker cannot speak. He also acknowledges his own limitations; any words he attributes to Walker must be of his own invention. Yet he says that he knows that Walker loves him, a reflection perhaps of his own love for Walker. And he knows that this is a bit of a fantasy, adding: "In my mind, we chat nonstop. But in actual life, my son can't speak" (p. 125).

All of these parents—Emily Rapp, Ian Brown, Savannah's mother, and Angie Lydicksen—are creating stories from their children's limited actions. They are aware there is very little evidence for their interpretations. Through their constant caregiving they become uniquely attuned, not only to their child's bodily needs, but also to their child's life narrative. It is important to note that, while the story is generated in the context of caregiving, it is not directly about caregiving. It is about establishing an identity within the family and a personhood that the rest of the world can understand. The parents become storytellers as an inevitable part of the act of caregiving. If there is no obvious story, they must perhaps invent one.

The question is: Whose story is this? Is it Walker's or his father's? Ronan's or his mother's? Since neither Walker nor Ronan can be cheated of his own story any more thoroughly than he has already been cheated by his disease, perhaps it does not matter. Yet Brown and Rapp remain the uncontested storytellers, and Walker's and Ronan's inner lives remain a mystery. I think it is likely that Walker and his father share their story, and that Ronan's story and his mother's are one and the same. Their lives, looped through the responsiveness needed to interpret needs, become a tangled thread, their stories inseparable.

With this in mind, the moral hazards of communication techniques like facilitated communication, where a caregiver can possibly direct the words being said by the child, become evident. Parents who desperately want to know their child's inner self must take extreme care when the possibility of a line of communication is opened in this way. It would be so tempting to produce the words a parent longs to hear and so difficult to dismiss them as fantasy. A responsive caregiver will continue to monitor the other cues to which they have become exquisitely sensitive, however. When they act on the new information received via facilitation, they will notice if their action causes any sign of physical or emotional distress. They must listen very carefully in order to remain open to alternative interpretations.

I do not wish to suggest that extreme caregiving parents are creating for their children false personalities or wronging their children through the stories they create. Quite the opposite, in fact. I maintain that caregiving without attention to narrative, to story, is incomplete. Clearly, the caregiver who treats the child merely as a body to be kept clean and fed is providing incomplete care. The parent who creates a story within the context of extreme caregiving, however improbable, is providing morally responsive care.

It is likely that the narrative created can benefit the parent as much, or more than, the child. Parents can find both reassurance and purpose in the story they tell themselves and others. Angie Lydicksen is probably not the only parent who, having no evidence otherwise, concludes that her child is happy. To believe that her son is happy must reassure her greatly and does not compromise his care in any way.

It is possible that the story can become a somewhat selfish form of disillusionment, provided only for the benefit of the parent. However, I believe that a caregiver's insistence on a certain story would be problematic only if the child seemed distressed by it. With their life stories so entangled, perhaps the making of stories in which the parents themselves find comfort is unavoidable. Bound by the daily necessities of caregiving, the life stories of extreme caregiver and cared-for become inseparable, their stories twined together and meeting the needs of both.

The Child as Teacher

In most situations, the creation of a life narrative by the caregiver is a form of responsiveness. Even if the story told cannot be proven true, a narrative created through attentive and competent caregiving becomes a valid part of the child's identity. We have seen, however, that many parents reject a narrative that identifies the child only by his diagnosis. In this section, I examine another commonly held identity story, one that is usually embraced by parents.

Severely ill children and children with disabilities are often described as being a teacher to everyone with whom they have had close contact. It is not unusual to hear that the child has taught parents and other adults lessons, often ones requiring a mature and complex wisdom. Very young children, and even infants, have been credited with teaching such things as dealing with adversity, bearing up under pain, or even revealing the meaning of life. Perhaps the parent has really learned these things by being a witness to the child's life, but that experience is related as a lesson, with the child placed in the position of teacher.

Parents of children with special needs are not alone in considering the person in need of care as a teacher; this idea comes up in academic literature as well. Arthur Frank (1995) discusses something he calls the "pedagogy of suffering," an idea that "one who suffers has something to teach"

(p. 150). The caregiver, as witness to the suffering of illness, learns important lessons from tending the wounded body. Some, like Frank, perceive this as a service received in return for the work of caregiving, thus equalizing the dependency of the relationship. Frank sees the sharing inherent in the caregiving relationship as a way to assuage loneliness and an opportunity for communion with others. I agree that life lessons can be learned by engaging another person with the responsiveness needed to perform moral caregiving.

But many children who require extreme care are nonverbal or minimally communicative and could not participate in this sort of communion. There are precedents for lessons taught without speech, however. One example comes from scientific researchers. One of the geneticists studying CFC who was interviewed by Brown (2011) makes the claim, "We are going to learn so much from these kids . . . . We are going to learn how to treat them better from knowing their genes . . . . We are going to learn so much about cancer treatment from these children" (p. 165). In this doctor's case, she's talking about medical information gleaned from studying children with CFC: specifically, information about the complicated connection between certain genetic defects in CFC that overlap with genes being studied as markers for cancer. These lessons will, of course, be learned from observations of the child's body—blood, bone marrow, and DNA—and not from the child's words and ideas. However, the child is given credit.

Christine Montross, in a book of meditations on the anatomy lab encountered in her first year of medical school, reports that a sort of learning relationship can be formed with even a dead body. As she explains in *Body of Work*, in some Thai Buddhist medical schools, the body to be dissected is given the title of "great teacher," held in high esteem, and honored in several ceremonies (2007, pp. 78–80). This is not standard practice in American medical schools, where measures are taken to distance the student from the humanity of the body. I know from experience there is a fair amount of emotional work that must be done by the student of anatomy to reconcile the knowledge received from this source with previously held notions of life and personhood. It may matter very much to the student whether the body in question is seen as a passive provider of cells and parts or a teacher of life lessons. The inert body obviously cannot actively participate in this process but still can be a respected source of teaching.

Based on their experience, the narrators of extreme caregiving stories are familiar with the idea that lessons learned can be taught by the most incommunicative of teachers. As Charles Hart, explains, people with autism taught him "what it means to be human, what it means to live in this baffling world of sights and sounds and messages." He goes on,

> Although their misunderstandings appear more obvious than my own, they have taught me never to underestimate the capacity of my fellow human beings to misunderstand or fail in communication. Most of all they have taught me that I can't assume that any two people think alike or that words will mean the same to the reader that they meant to the writer. (1989, p. 258)

Like Kittay, he acknowledges that all of us "see each other through a glass darkly" (2011, p. 614). No matter how well we communicate, in words or in writing, there is always the possibility of misunderstanding. He thanks both his autistic brother and son for this lesson, though it was likely learned through his own thoughtful and empathetic listening.

Shelly Greenhaw, mother of a non-verbal child with CFC, in an interview with Ian Brown, explains how her daughter, Kinley has taught her:

> Right now, I think Kinley has—oh boy—without trying, taught me how to live with joy, despite tough circumstances. And to use my time wisely. Not to worry about tomorrow too much, but to enjoy today. She's taught me to laugh at the little things. She's helped me with my vision of life. Boy, she's helped me see that each person has something to contribute, and to learn from as many people as we can . . . . I think I've learned, too, that we're very interdependent. (Brown, 2011, pp. 144–145)

Kinley is no more able to communicate verbally than is Brown's son, Walker. Her mother admits that teaching is not something Kinley is trying to do, but she still identifies her daughter as the source of her learning.

The lessons taught by these children often are important ones: lessons in philosophy and humanity and love. They provide lessons in personal growth. Priscilla Gilman, whose son has mild autism, writes: "the blessings of being his mother far outweigh the worry and stress and fatigue. Truly he has made me an infinitely stronger, more patient and compassionate person" (2011, pp. 196–197). They provide lessons in compassion and understanding of disability. Ian Brown writes, "The disabled are a challenge to everyone's established sense of order: they frighten us, if not with their faces, then with their obvious need. They call us to be more than we ever thought we would have to be" (2011, p.150). Or they can teach us that something we once thought important is not so critical after all. "We didn't yet realize how much she would teach us," Kittay writes of her daughter, "but we already knew that we had learned something. That which we believed we valued, what we—I—thought was at the center of humanity, the capacity for thought, for reason, was not it, not it at all" (1999, p. 150).

But perhaps the most important lesson taught (or learned) is how, simply, to just "be," or "to live in the moment," as the now-ubiquitous cliché has it. Ian Brown (2011) reports that a developmental pediatrician, who had just diagnosed significant delays in his son Walker, told him this: "The Buddhists say the way to enlightenment, to pure being, is by getting your mind out of the way. I'm not trying to be trite, but Walker already knows how to do that. He is pure being. He may be developmentally delayed, or moderately retarded, but in that way, he's already miles ahead of most of us" (p. 68). Presumably this specialist knew many children with developmental delays. Possibly he had told other parents this in the past. Walker was less than a year old when he reached this stage of enlightenment. Brown, whose response to platitudes is usually tinged with cynicism, accepts this completely, adding, "That was the first time someone suggested Walker had a gift the rest of us didn't" (p. 68).

It is important to remember that none of these children can communicate verbally. Yet their parents are certainly learning lessons in philosophy and humanity and the value of life. I believe that the teaching is occurring in the context of responsive caregiving. The parent learns these things by listening intently to the child's needs and remaining open to the small clues by which the child's identity can be discerned. Perhaps the moral work of putting aside one's own needs and learning to interpret the needs of someone who is voiceless is itself a source of enlightenment. However, many narrators also claim this teaching as a demonstration of the value of the child's life.

Brown expounds on his lessons from Walker later in his book: "[O]n his good days, Walker is proof of what the imperfect and the fragile have to offer; a reminder that there are many ways to be human; a concentrator of joy; an insistent nudge to pay attention to every passing mote of daily life that otherwise slips by uncounted" (p. 180). But his wife disagrees with him, resenting the well-worn concept that his disability might supply others with some special understanding. She is quite bitter about it, saying, "I'm not sure that I agree that his lasting value is to have touched people. That his whole life has to be this fucking Gandhi thing, making people feel better about themselves . . . . I think his life should have a value of its own" (p. 182).

Emily Rapp stands with Brown's wife. She too has heard the platitudes that the disabled have lessons to teach us all, and clearly disagrees with them.

> The meaning of Ronan's life was not to teach me; we often say this about people who defy our notions of normal and I find it pathetic, patronizing, and a way of distancing ourselves from our own fragile bodies and tenuous lives. I don't believe that disabled people exist to teach people life stories—that is not their purpose; it isn't anyone's purpose. We are not "the disabled," some shapeless, teeming mass of nonnormative bodies designed for teaching purposes, like some kind of specially designed pedagogical barbarian horde. (2013, p. 114)

I too am uncomfortable with the idea of people with disabilities as a source of enlightenment, and I support Emily Rapp's and Johanna Brown's position. If there are lessons to be sought, we must learn them for ourselves and not expect children with disabilities, or their parents, to provide them.

As Rapp points out, we are doing people with disabilities a disservice if we think of them merely as tools for our own learning. Believing without justification that we understand what it is like to be another person is not a sense of responsiveness. When we create the narrative of the child as the teacher, we create for the child a story that is not her own and functions mainly to reassure the parent and the outside world. This is hardly responding to the needs of the child—as we ought to—it is responding to the need of the outside world to grasp some clear justification for the child's existence.

Expecting parents to maintain the fiction that the child is a gifted teacher for us seems to me a particularly unfair way to enforce a societal standard that bases value on ability. We have seen that one of the responsibilities of being an extreme caregiver is to establish and maintain social value for the child. This particular method attempts to equalize the lack of some skills by claiming a different, and overlooked, skill, which is possessed only by the child with disabilities. This actually serves to uphold the faulty premise that value and acceptance must be based on ability. We should not have to make our children into angels so they can gain acceptance or value.

However my biggest reason for objecting to the child-as-teacher myth is that it underplays and negates the value of caregiving. I believe that learning is a product of the personal journey that is extreme caregiving.

Any teaching is not actively provided by the child but actively attained by the parent as a product of responsive caregiving. If we claim that the benefits come from the child, we miss the value of the complex work these parents are doing. We miss the possibility that, along with the long hours and sleepless nights, the constant meeting of the bodily and emotional needs of a child by responsive caregiving is an act of creation and beauty. Sometimes it enriches the parent as well as the child.

Ian Brown, after writing about arguments with his wife and daughter Hayley, describes a good morning with his family:

> But there are other times too—moments of unstoppable pleasure . . . . This is something, you see: every time [Walker] is happy, he is as happy as he has ever been. Hayley, a delicate and skilled ballet dancer, twisting with Walker to music on the stereo, Walker on the moon with joy. Minutes from his life. Everyday occurrences for a normal child. But I know their true value. (2011, pp. 66–67)

Brown has learned the value of simple joy. He suspects that parents with "a normal child" have more of these moments, but I am not convinced this is so, since those hypothetical parents might not be as well-equipped to recognize them.

Almost every parent narrative attempts to convey the lessons learned from caring for their child. Though stated in a variety of ways—from learning how to slow down to how to love without reservation—all the lessons come very close to the theme of learning to live by a new set of values. Parents must, sometimes by necessity, abandon the societal rules that place material wealth and achievements in one's career as the primary measurements of value and success. Instead, they measure success in terms of the capacity for love embodied in the giving and receiving of care.

In a recent political science book, *Caring Democracy*, Joan Tronto suggested that a democratic society might run better if the accumulation of wealth was not its first priority. Instead, she recommends that the provision of care should be moved from its current position of invisibility to the center of all democratic decisions. She writes,

> We have got things backwards now. The key to living well, for all people, is to live a care-filled life, a life in which one is well cared for by others when one needs it, cares well for oneself, and has room to provide for the caring—for other people, animals, institutions, and ideals—that gives one's life its particular meaning. A truly free society makes people free to care.

> A truly equal society gives people equal chances to be well cared for, and to engage in caring relationships. —(2013, p. 170)

The parents who are doing extreme caregiving have already learned the value of caring itself, the rewards that come from stepping outside the usual measurements of success. Their job is made much harder, though, by a lack of equality accorded in the distribution of care resources. Care itself is distributed according to wealth rather than need, and those who take on care often take on a too-large burden.

If we could acknowledge the lesson learned by extreme caregiving, we might be able to envision a different kind of society, one that understands that we all depend to a large extent on others. Lacking this understanding we have become a society where we ignore care and make life decisions according to a utilitarian equation where ability is everything. But if we could learn the value of care, we could become a different sort of moral community, one where we acknowledge our interdependence and provide help to those who need it whether or not we can ascribe to them a value based on contribution or potential contribution to the economy. This, I believe, is the lesson that extreme caregivers have learned.

The child has not chosen the role of teacher and may be completely unaware of it. That the child is a teacher of otherwise inaccessible mysteries and profound truths is a story imposed on him by others. Though we might learn something from Walker and Ronan and Ted, they should not be expected to perform as our teachers. However, we can learn by careful observation and by participating in the care of the child. We can bear witness to both suffering and the tenacity of life. We can, by cultivating the quiet patience needed to attend to a child whose ability to respond is minimal, perhaps add something to our own stories. We can learn how to "live a care-filled life" and to value interdependent and caring relationships. It is the parents performing extreme caregiving who have this lesson to teach us.

Letting Go

I introduced Jeanette, the little girl who survived near-drowning in a backyard swimming pool, in Chapter 5, as an example of the emotional burden that can be carried by parents. There are children like Jeanette in every pediatric hospital I have ever been in. They are the survivors of head trauma, neonatal strokes, severe genetic syndromes, overwhelming meningitis, and extreme prematurity, to name just a few. They are tube-fed and often trach-dependent. Some of them have been at home under their parents' care for a decade or more. The oldest I know of has been in a persistent vegetative state since she was in an automobile accident as a teenager. She is in her thirties.

When Jeanette arrived at my hospital years ago, I briefly considered the emotional burden that might have caused her father to be so uncooperative. In these pages, I considered the likelihood that the emotional burden of Jeanette's life for her family was different than it was for me. Though I could not look into Jeanette's own story, I have no doubt that Jeanette's family, along with every one of those parents of children in ICUs across the country, could tell you who their child is as a person, their likes and dislikes, moods and quirks, all filtered through the story they have created while anticipating and fulfilling their needs.

But at some point, all will reach a time when medicine is only barely able to keep the child alive. This was not yet the case for Jeanette, but it had only been eighteen months since her accident. Despite the best care, these children begin getting pneumonia or other infections that become increasingly resistant to antibiotics. Some of them survive multiple cardiac arrests or multiple life-saving surgeries. They can spend years deteriorating, in and out of the ICU, on ventilators, dialysis, intravenous feedings, and esoteric drips.

For hospital staff, these lives often seem untenable, and repeatedly saving them a cruelty rather than a mercy. Indeed, there comes a time when it might be appropriate to let the child go, in order to finally end the child's suffering. In this era of "shared decision-making," where physician and parent are supposed collaborate in the child's care, we often seek permission from the parents to withdraw aggressive medical treatment. Parents asked to make this difficult decision are often inundated by medical information, as if clinicians assume that the narrative composed from their medical knowledge and the information on the child's chart is the only story of the child's life. Parents who resist this are thought to either lack understanding of medicine or have unrealistic, or possibly selfish, attitudes overwhelmed by emotion.

Yet, in framing the decision in this way, we are essentially asking parents to accept a new and different identity for their child, one that is crafted, not from the experience of living with the child, but from the child's medical record. It might require that they accept that the child's life is composed mostly of suffering or that no child would "want to live like this." But the child has been living at home under care that is very little different from that in the hospital, often for years. That has become the new normal for the family.

Sometimes we say that the parents are "not ready" to let go. Deanna Fei, whose daughter was born at 23 weeks, experienced several times when it seemed likely that her daughter would die. Even she thought that because her daughter was so sick, letting her go might be easy. At one point a neonatologist called to warn her that her daughter's condition had worsened and attempted to prepare her for her daughter's death. She writes a litany of the things she thought she was supposed to be thinking in order to accept her daughter's death:

No matter what I've told myself, I'm not prepared.
I don't know her yet.
She's not really a baby.
I love her, but not the way I love my son.
If she doesn't make it, it's for the best.
If there ever was a time when these terrible lies would have made it easier to let her go, that time is past. I know this now. My daughter has claimed her small, dark, turbulent corner of this world, and despite the wall I've tried to build between us, that's where I live too. (Fei, 2015, pp. 116–117)

Her daughter was only a few days old at this point, and already the attachment was undeniable. Despite the fact that Fei was not expecting her child for another several months, and that she had never been able to physically hold her, their stories were already entwined. The way in which she was holding her daughter was different, not only from what the neonatologists seemed to believe, but also from what she herself expected it to be. No matter what she told herself, she was not ready. Perhaps no one can be ready.

No matter how much care the child needs, the parent in turn needs the child. Death will not seem like the laying down of a terrible burden. It may be "dark and turbulent," but the child has claimed her corner of the world, and that is where the parents live also. The stories of parent and child are interwoven and inseparable. Yet I do not believe that the inseparability of their stories results in lack of objectivity that interferes with the parents' ability to determine the best interests of their child. I do not believe that parents selfishly extend their children's lives for their own benefit. They are holding their children to the best of their ability. But sometimes it is time to let go.

We must not forget that every child, even in infancy and regardless of their impairments, is already a complex person within a family. The family has been holding the child in an identity within the family, telling stories that often began before the child was born. If they give permission to withdraw care, they will have to tell a new story about their care. They will also have to learn to hold that child in a new way, in memory (Lindemann, 2014).

We must understand the caregiving relationship between parent and child when we approach the subject of withdrawal of aggressive care. Until we understand the story of who the child is in his parents' world, recognizing both the burdens and benefits of care, it will be impossible to adequately support parents in a decision to allow their child's life to end. That understanding starts with recognizing the moral consequences of responsive caregiving and the ways in which the lives of parent and child are bound together. Perhaps we, too, as responsive caregivers, must begin by asking, not just how the child feels, but also who the child is. And we must accept the answers, not as a tragic denial or delusion, but as truth.

Moral caregiving requires responsiveness to care. The caregiver must retain an openness to the care-receiver, a responsiveness that is, at its best, a form of mutual storytelling. The feedback between caregiver and cared-for creates a relationship between them, which allows the care-receiver dignity and personhood despite dependency, and the caregiver a sense of connection and, possibly, self-worth.

I have said that this mutual storytelling is more difficult when the care-receiver is unable to provide a reliable response. For a child whose disabilities include limited verbal communication, the caregiver is in a position of uncertainty. Extreme caregivers whose children are, and will always remain, minimally responsive must by necessity uphold both sides of the responsiveness feedback loop. These parents are called on, essentially, to provide the responses to care that their child cannot. Over a lifetime, they might find it particularly difficult to "hold well" the life story of their child. It may even be possible for the caregiving relationship to create and maintain a person who does not exist or who no longer exists. This is precarious territory and immensely increases the moral and emotional work that must be performed by parent extreme caregivers.

As professionals, we must be aware of the existence and importance of the relationship the parent is creating. Those who fail to understand this relationship might be tempted to see caring for a child with multiple complex needs as an unmitigated burden. They might envision placement in an institution, or even death, as an immense relief, the laying down of burdensome care. As a society, we have encouraged parents to raise children with disabilities as valued persons, but there are seemingly still limits to our willingness to support them.

I have shown that extreme caregivers spend a good deal of emotional effort attempting to read their child's limited responses. They become finely tuned to the messages of discomfort or wellness read sometimes only from their children's bodies. Indeed, they are expected by the medical system to do this as an adjunct to providing competent home care, though they reject the medical diagnosis as the whole identity of the child. Instead they interpret their childrens' moods and personality along with their physical bodily needs. They attempt to create larger meaning from their child's responses. Sometimes the response they receive is barely perceptible to an outside observer. And sometimes parents and observers alike transfer some of their own longing for a response to the child, by envisioning him as the active teacher of the life lessons they have learned from the experience of caregiving.

The result is the creation of a story of a life that might be at least partly imaginary. This story is perhaps an attempt to create hope in the face of disability or a buffer against the endless tedium of providing bodily care. At the end of life, it may be difficult to recognize the moment when all hope of a new response is gone, and when that part of the story is over. Nonetheless, the story emerges from the responsiveness that I believe is required for moral caregiving. I believe that it is a commendable, desirable, and perhaps unavoidable, element of good caregiving, and it should be encouraged and nurtured.

For the most part, I think the story created is mutually beneficial, creating a bond between caregiver and cared-for that acknowledges both of them as persons of importance in the world, despite limited levels of communication. Ian Brown speaks to his son by clicking his tongue. Or, rather, when Brown clicks at Walker, sometimes Walker clicks back. It is not much of a clue to Walker's feelings; the clicks are only noises they make at each other. But they are not without meaning. Brown writes,

> My relationship with Walker, after all, had been personal, and private; we operated by our own standards, by what worked between us. I "spoke" to him and he "spoke" to me, clicking our tongues back and forth to one another to let each other know that we were paying attention, that we knew the other was there, and listening. (2011, p. 159)

Brown and his son are listening to each other, creating a world together, in which both of them can function. It is no less important than any other relationship between parent and child. This responsiveness seems to me to be the heart of extreme caregiving and, in fact, of any caregiving. It seems a good standard to set for responsiveness; to know that someone is paying attention; that someone else is there and listening.

In the next chapter, I consider a different aspect of letting go: finding a place for the child to move on. It is a difficult step, and not just because there are so few options for placement. The parent must risk opening their private world and letting others in. They must allow someone else to take over part of the child's story and be open to the things other responsive listeners might find out about him. As we shall see, this can be of enormous benefit to both parent and child.

CHAPTER 8 | Holding the Future

I GOT MY first uncomfortable glimpse of my brother's future at our family dinner table in the spring of 1971, the year I started to plan for college. We still had family dinners back then, every night, eating all together around the kitchen table. My mother sat at the end of the table, nearest to the stove, and next to my brother Paul so that she could help him with his food, if need be. I sat on her left, across from Paul. My other brother sat next to me; my grandmother, father, and sister sat at the other end.

Paul by that time didn't need to be fed anymore. He used a fork and spoon, though my mother sometimes had to cut things up for him. I'm pretty sure he was able to chew with his mouth closed, but I had actually stopped watching him during the days when he hadn't. He would have been about eleven.

We always talked as we ate, about school or current events or the project my father was working on at his lab. We would complain about how much food cost, whether someone really needed new shoes, or the amusing behavior of that odd history teacher. It didn't matter. There was only one rule. My brother Paul didn't say much, but if he did, all other conversation would cease immediately while we tried to figure out what he was saying. It went something like this:

"Ahhhh . . ." Paul would say. He always started with this, as though he had to first find his voice and then slowly shape words around it. Meanwhile whatever anyone else had been about to say was forgotten.

"Ahhh . . . movie projectors go around and around." This was fairly typical. He adored movie projectors. He still does.

At this point, the person who had been trying to say something interesting might try to stop it by saying something like, "Yes, we know that. Now about that history . . ." But they wouldn't get very far.

My mother would say, brightly, "Did you see a movie in school?" to Paul.

"Ahhh . . . yes."

"What was it about?"

Silence.

"Was it about trains?"

Confused stare.

"Did you like it?"

"Ahhh . . . movie projectors go around and around." This would be said in a louder, unhappy voice, the way you would express frustration at an audience that failed to understand your point. Movies were never the point. Movie projectors, on the other hand, were endlessly fascinating.

I found this whole process immensely irritating.

That night the subject was a summer trip to visit colleges. I needed to select the colleges I wished to apply to. My parents were hoping that my sister would begin to show more interest in colleges other than the one her boyfriend wanted to go to. Even my other brother, Paul's twin, was thinking about where he might like to go.

Paul said, "Ahhh . . ."

We stopped talking. I feigned patience. But Paul did not say anything about projectors. It was worse than that. Much worse.

He said, "Ahhh . . . I go a college too."

There was a massive silence. My heart sank down to a place where it began to be digested along with my dinner. It was clearly, blatantly, devastatingly obvious that Paul was never going to do any such thing. I put my fork down, feeling suddenly defeated, as the awful implications of Paul's future closed in.

Paul had always wanted to do everything the rest of us did. We always let him. If he did not do it well, we pretended not to notice. His attempt would be met with lavish praise, often more than was forthcoming for our obviously superior attempts. Of course, Paul would want to go to college too.

When Paul was eighteen months old, he had been diagnosed as "mentally retarded." Doctors told my mother that he would never walk or talk. We had, over the years, made a sort of family project out of proving them wrong. We were aided in this endeavor by our schools. Paul attended something called sixth grade, though he and his classmates were actually busily and repeatedly failing kindergarten. It to me felt like a social game, played with words and diminished expectations.

But college was not a game. We couldn't pretend our way around it. Paul could barely count to twenty. He could read only about forty words, most of which were logos for fast food places. It took him five minutes to write his name. There was no way in hell that Paul was ever going to college. In fact, horrifyingly, there were a lot more things that Paul was never going to do. The immensity of them floored me.

But, into the silence, my mother said, cheerfully, "No, Paul. You're not going to college." She said this without apparent regret, in a matter-of-fact way that was only a little bit forced, as though she truly believed that college was an option easily discarded, and not, as she'd told me repeatedly, the only gateway to an adequate life. Then she continued, firmly, "You're going to be a working man." Her cheerful reasonableness made it clear that being a working man was something to be immensely proud of.

Paul nodded. He said, "Ahh . . . I a working man," patting himself with an open palm to his chest and smiling broadly. Even now, forty years later, if you ask him what he does, he gives the same answer, with the same smile and evident pride.

I was relieved—and astonished. It was good to know that my parents did not actually expect Paul to go to college. The disaster of arguing about his disability in front of him had been averted. But the pat answer my mother had provided was full of flaws and raised questions about Paul's future that could not even be asked at that point. The astonishing thing was that my mother knew—had known all along—that the game we were playing did not end in a fully functional and independent future. That she'd been prepared for this, with a practiced statement about being a "working man," whatever that meant, was almost a betrayal.

I had been so caught up in my own adolescent concerns that I had not thought about Paul's future. I had not done the simple math of my brother's development and ended up with the obvious conclusion. My parents, of course, had. At eleven, Paul was functioning as a very slow five-year-old. Even if he continued to progress, he would not reach high school, let alone college. He would not read Aristotle or *To Kill a Mockingbird* or the newspaper. He would not learn algebra or long division, or even be able to make change for a dollar. As for being a "working man," I could not imagine him as a plumber or truck driver. He was strong, but his poor balance and motor control made even moving boxes beyond him. I had no idea what my mother had in mind. Yet she seemed to think that this goal, possibly just as farfetched as college, was totally within reach.

But all that was shadowed by the biggest realization: Paul would never be able to live without supervision. My parents would age, but Paul would never be able to move out. From that point, as I plotted my own future, I always had, way in the back of my mind, a contingency plan for where Paul would stay, if he had to move in with me. I don't know when my sister and other brother came to the same conclusion, but they eventually developed contingency plans too.

That we have not yet needed to activate our contingency plans is a credit to the hard work done by my parents and other advocates for change. We were also immensely lucky. Paul has indeed become a working man, by his own definition, at a sheltered workshop. He moved out at age thirty and has a new family at his group home. He has become a Special Olympics swimmer and, at age fifty-two, an Eagle Scout. Obtaining these things for him was not easy and is in no way assured to the children growing up today with similar disabilities. The rest of this chapter outlines the problems that still exist and explores the key components of a successful future suggested by caring theory developed from Tronto's phases of care (Tronto, 1993) and from the work of Jean Vanier, a pioneer in caring for adults with mental handicaps (Spink, 1991.

Preparing for the Future

The recognition that their child's disabilities might limit their choice of futures comes to different families at different times and in a multitude of ways. I have not fully researched this moment of discovery, but I believe that for many it begins at the time of diagnosis. Beth Price, the mother of a newborn with Down syndrome writes,

> Even though we were weeks from bringing Jude home from the hospital, I was already wondering about whether he would ever be capable of leaving, of living on his own someday. Parents work hard for almost two decades to try and instill everything they think their children will need to fly when it is time to leave the nest. But would Jude ever enjoy any independence? It bothered me to think about my husband and me never being alone again. (2007, pp. 189–190)

As the work of many parent narrators demonstrates, parents of children with Down syndrome begin to think (and worry) about their children's future dependency early. However, in their essays, including the one quoted above, many such parents come to the conclusion that those worries are incorrect because they are based on societal impressions that devalue people with Down syndrome. By the time her son Jude is eighteen months old, Price's worries seem to have lessened. She continues, "I wish I had known when Jude was born all that I know now about the bright future that is within reach for him" (p. 191).

There is indeed a bright future available, but it is not the same as the one most parents imagine before their child is diagnosed. Most of the parent memoirs recognize this and wrestle with the new definition of achievement. Most of them also end on a positive note, with a child in their toddler years, advancing faster than the dire predictions that came from the medical profession. The children with Down syndrome exhibiting a bright future in the essay collection *Gifts*, are only several months to several years old; the oldest is in eighth grade. The reality is that most of the sixty-five children with Down syndrome whose parents wrote essays about them will not live independently. Like my brother Paul, they will grow up and learn things that surprise everyone, but life without supervision will never be possible. These parents have not yet begun the part of the journey where they must continue their love and support into adulthood. Nor have they taken into account the fact that, when their child grows up, they, too, will be twenty years older.

A study of quality of life of adults with "mental retardation or developmental disabilities" (MR/DD), published in 2001, states the problem even more boldly: "One unique aspect of the quality of life of adults with MR/DD who live at home with their parents is the impermanence of this caregiving arrangement and the concomitant need for planning for future care and quality of life after the parent is no longer the primary caregiver" (Seltzer & Krauss, 2001, p. 110). Even if the parent can persist in caregiving for an MR/DD child into adulthood, it is not a permanent solution. As parents age or develop care needs of their own, the arrangement becomes less reliable. The researchers felt that the insecurity of the living arrangement could have a negative effect on the MR/DD person's quality of life. I suspect that it also has a negative effect on the caregiver's quality of life, and that the worry continues as a thread over the child's entire life.

When his son with Down syndrome was six years old, Michael Berube wrote, "Jamie has come a very long way since the days he spent supine in the NICU. He also has a very, very long way to go." According to Berube, Jamie had yet to learn how to dress himself and use the toilet. He had yet to cope with the teenage years, or begin to seek opportunities for living independently or finding employment. Berube continues, "And then, when he's thirty or forty, we can begin to worry about the incidence of Alzheimer's in Down syndrome, and we can agonize over which scenario might bring us more emotional pain: the thought of our outliving him, or the thought of him outliving us" (1996, p. 261).

The few parents who continued to write about their children with developmental delays into their teenage years, all faced this issue. The essential impossibility of taking care of a child they expect and hope will outlive them looms large. Their narratives contain multiple statements like this one from Ian Brown. He and his wife agree that it doesn't matter where their son Walker lives, "*As long as someone loves him every day.*" Then they ask, "Who will that be? That is the question . . . as much as I think about getting through the days with Walker, I think more about the future. Who will care for Walker after we are dead?" (2011, p. 184).

Those worries are there, as a thread that becomes more visible during the darker times—the setbacks and the sleepless nights. Brown acknowledges that the future is an ongoing worry and reports that this is so, also, for all the families of children with the same syndrome as Walker that he has met. Berube talks about the worry as something that will catch up to him when his son is older, but he obviously is fully aware of it much earlier. He clearly understands, when his son is six years old, that Jamie's future independence, happiness, and self-esteem are not guaranteed and will require extra work in order to be accomplished.

The options for meeting the needs of an intellectually disabled child into adulthood have improved somewhat over time, as both knowledge about intellectual disability and social supports have advanced. But the problem of long-term care is far from solved. Decades of improvements have increased the potential for development for multitudes of children with disabilities, but there will always be some for whom independent living, or even living in group homes, is not possible. Many of those children have not moved out of their parents' care.

Jack, who has severe autism, still lives with his parents. He does not talk and still has toileting accidents at age twenty-eight. Jack is allowed to wander around the house, self-stimming whenever he needs to. His parents and a long-term home care aide make sure he does nothing to endanger himself, like wander away or forget to eat. They all are exquisitely attuned to his moods and watch him closely for signs of agitation that might lead to a meltdown. Fortunately, there are very few of these, but at 265 pounds, he has caused injuries. His parents are in their sixties; even the home care aide is in his fifties. They know that there is a limit to the time when they can provide care, but they also know that there are few people who know Jack as well as they do and could provide an environment where he is both safe and happy.

According to a study from 2001, Jack and his parents are not alone. Statistics showed that 60% of the 3.35 million people with MR/DD were living with family caregivers, most often their parents. (This number included all ages and a wide range of level of disability.) The researchers estimated there were about a half-million people with intellectual disabilities in the United States living in a variety of supported residential settings including group homes, foster care, nursing homes, and institutions. A slightly larger number were living with parents over the age of sixty (Braddock, et al, 2001). I doubt that the numbers have changed much in the last decade.

It is tempting to try to estimate the number of adults with MR/DD still living at home based on the number of people on wait lists for group homes, since this is the hoped-for destination for many young adults with intellectual disabilities. However, there are numerous programs, through equally numerous agencies, which vary on a state-by-state basis. Many states have separate wait lists for placement and for the financial services that might make placement possible. Some parents have listed their dependent adult children on wait lists at more than one agency or institution. However, researchers report that over half of adults with MR/DD still living at home are not on any wait list. Up to 20% have done no planning for the future at all (Seltzer & Krauss, 2001). I can imagine a variety of reasons for this, including an impression, not always inaccurate, that they can do a better job at home and an equally correct assumption that services are difficult to obtain. Indeed, though families in crisis can usually be given fairly rapid priority placement, national availability of residential services is inadequate to meet the growing need (Braddock, 2001).

The number of people on waiting lists for out-of-home placement is appalling. In Kansas, an activist group called End the Wait Kansas, has determined that there are almost 5,000 people with intellectual disabilities on the Department of Health and Human Services wait list for services, including group home placement (O'Higgins, 2011). And a 2013 article in the *New Jersey Star-Ledger* reported that there were about 8,000 people with intellectual disabilities including autism waiting for placement in New Jersey. The article reports that a Special Needs Housing Trust had been established earlier, but after $168 million in funding and six years, only 1,500 new spots had been created (Goldberg, 2011).

My rather personal and imprecise experience comes from suburban Philadelphia. In the late 1980s, my parents, then in their sixties, were unable to find a home for Paul, my dependent thirty-year-old brother. They had some experience in political activism, working with the Montgomery

County Association for Retarded Children when my brother was a child. They found a state senator who expressed interest in the problem of group home placement and was willing to attend a meeting. ("Aren't there group homes?" he asked. "Yes," my mother reportedly replied; "And the only way I can get my son into one is by dying.") My parents relied on nothing but word-of-mouth contact (there was no internet) and had only a few weeks to inform their fellow caregivers. There were almost 300 people at that meeting, all in their late fifties or sixties, living with a middle-aged "child" in the same small county on the edge of Philadelphia.

Another paper, from Canada, reports that many families lacked "permanency planning," or a plan for meeting the residential, legal, and financial needs of their child once they were no longer able to do so. Uncertainty about who would provide care for their child in the future was a large concern among older parents living with their adult intellectually disabled child. Efforts are being made to aid these parents in planning for the future (Weeks et al., 2009). I suspect that without a societal commitment to creating more residential placement opportunities and providing ongoing financial support, permanency planning might look more like a wish list than an actual plan.

The future becomes one of the many uncertain things to which families doing extreme caregiving must be attentive. There is, of course, the possibility that the developmentally delayed child will catch up with his peers and be able to live independently. But in the frequent circumstances when that does not happen, parents must, with very little support, carve out a place for their child to thrive beyond the time that they can provide care.

But what is it that parents want for their intellectually delayed child in adulthood? Josh Greenfeld gave this answer when Noah was twelve years old, and the family was desperately trying to find a place where he could live. Greenfeld wrote:

> What do I want for Noah? I want a residence. I want a humane situation, small, life-sized, without a massive bureaucracy hovering over it. I want people caring for him who are dedicated rather than money motivated. I don't know where one can find such people these days . . . (1986, p. 78)

At that point, years of behavior modification therapy had failed to teach Noah to talk or behave appropriately, and he was becoming increasingly destructive and impossible to handle. Noah had been through several trials of residential therapy, all with unfortunate outcomes. One program was terminated after evidence of abuse. His father's expectations weren't very high. All he wanted was a place that he could afford, where Noah would be cared for in a humane way.

Today parents' expectations can be much higher. In 1996, Michael Berube wanted much more for his son with Down syndrome. He imagined that, as an adult, his son, Jamie

> would become an individual little human, and perhaps someday he would even achieve the kind of individual autonomy that's been prized in the Western world, since the eighteenth century or thereabouts, as the philosophical foundation for political and ethical action, but he would achieve these things partly by modeling, partly with a little help from his friends. If he were to walk and talk like the rest of the semi-autonomous individuals in his peer groups, at age two or at twenty-two, he would need a lot of support. He would realize his individual potential only by leaning on our mutual human interdependence—just like everyone else, only a bit more so. (p. 176)

In 2011, Ian Brown, after traveling extensively to witness the types of care possible for his son, wrote:

> I wanted to see if there was a graceful, meaningful way for Walker to live in this world—to see for myself if it was possible to create, not just an ad hoc solution to his needs, but a community and family he might call his own, even—this was the most radical notion—a liberty and freedom he could claim. (p. 226)

Berube and Brown want something very similar for their sons, despite the differences in Jamie's and Walker's abilities. Like the developmental progress adapted to a quieter, slower scale of success, the goals for the future also have to be reimagined. They want their sons to be treated as individuals with grace and meaning, whose full potential can be reached with support. They want their sons to be part of a community and family, and claim as much freedom and independence as possible. Berube in addition acknowledges that we all require some support from others, and that his son, in his need for help, is just like everyone else. We are all in fact dependent on each other.

In a practical sense, parents looking for placement out of the home for their child, I believe, are looking for someone to provide, not only physical care, but also emotionally responsive care. Of course, the caregiving situation has to be able to monitor health, provide appropriate medical care, and assist as needed in the physical activities of daily living. But parents can hope that a new person or group of people will interact positively with the child, creating and holding them in an identity based on the work already done by the family. It is even possible that a responsive caregiver might be able to expand the possibilities for the identity already established by the family, just as happens when any child finally leaves their first home.

Jean Vanier was a pioneer in caring for adults with intellectual disabilities, beginning in 1964, when my brother was four years old, by inviting three mentally challenged men to live with him. He got more competent at this over the years, and his communities for the mentally disabled, called L'Arche, now exist across the world. Both Ian Brown and Michael Berube are aware of Vanier's work, and Brown wrote about his visit to the first L'Arche community, in Trosley-Breuil, France, in his book *The Boy in the Moon*. Brown reports that his son will unfortunately never be able to live in a L'Arche community, as the wait list is twenty years long (2011, p. 187).

I cannot agree with all of Vanier's philosophy. I do not share his opinion that mentally handicapped people possess a "spiritual openness" and a special "place in the heart of God" (Spink, 1991, p. 34). Like the assertion that handicapped children are our teachers (see Chapter 7), this attempts to assign value based on the possession of a special knowledge. I also am a bit uncomfortable with his "call" to care for the mentally handicapped, which he described as hearing "the 'primal cry of people with handicaps,' a cry which expresses in their very flesh a yearning for friendship combined with a sense of being unworthy and the doubt that anyone could ever want them" (Spink, 1991, p. 38). I am suspicious of the religious origins of these supposed feelings of unworthiness and self-doubt. Ian Brown also took exception to these ideas, particularly Jean Vanier's statement that a morally advanced person should "see the face of God within the disabled" who "bring us closer to God." Brown responds, "I wish I could believe in Vanier's God. But the truth is, I do not see the face of the Almighty in Walker. Instead, I see the face of my boy; I see what is human, and lively and flawed at once. Walker is no saint and neither am I" (2011, p. 284).

Nonetheless, Vanier's L'Arche communities have been steadily working their way toward something desirable and enormously beautiful. In his communities, mentally handicapped people live side-by-side with their caregivers and essentially care for each other. In her biography of Vanier, Kathryn Spink (1991) describes this "special relationship of reciprocity which remains at the very heart of L'Arche" (p. 44). She says that Vanier "wanted to create a family around them, a place where they could grow in all the dimensions of their being. They began to get to know each other, to learn how to live together, to care for one another, to have fun and to pray together" (p. 41). The people living together in each house do chores together, eat together, and enjoy each other's company, to the best of everyone's ability.

The philosophy of L'Arche includes not only establishing a home for the mentally handicapped but also a workplace, as a second component necessary for living. They believe that a separate place, a workshop, preferably in a different location from the home, is desirable, even for the most minimally functional of persons.

> Work had to be found of a kind that would allow mentally handicapped people to develop their particular gifts and give them access to the dignity of a salary, no matter how small. There was an unmistakable happiness that sprang from a handicapped person's discovery that he or she could make something beautiful or useful. (Spink, 1991, p. 50)

The work area becomes another place where meaning and purpose can be found. It is not necessary to discover great artistic talent or even any particular skill. The important part is the freedom to leave the home during the day to make some contribution, no matter how small, to the world.

A third component of this graceful living is community involvement. In the early stages, L'Arche expanded quickly and dramatically, and was in danger of taking over an area, making it an isolated spot where only the handicapped and their caregivers were present. To avoid becoming isolated from the larger world, later L'Arche houses sought integration into the local community, including adapting to religions other than Catholicism and accepting secular growth. In part by necessity, L'Arche also works with and for government and charitable agencies to provide for their resident's needs.

The grace, meaning, and supported autonomy desired by Brown and Berube and, really, all parents of any child, are found in these three components. We want our kids to find a new home, where new people will "love them every day," and take over the job of cultivating them as the best person possible. We want them to find work that they enjoy and find meaningful. And we want them to be part of the world, with friendships and hobbies and relationships with people who are not their parents.

All three of these things have been influential in my brother's life, and, in many cases are, I think, exemplary in the way they have been carried out. I will discuss each of these components separately, in the order in which they appeared in his life. First, oddly, was meaningful work, growing out of a summer day program sponsored by the county Association for Retarded Children. Next was community involvement, brought about by the efforts of a Presbyterian church that sponsored social events; the Special Olympics where he won medals for swimming; and the Boy Scouts of America, which chartered a troop for boys with special needs. The last to arrive, at age thirty, was a new place to live, a way to move out and move on. Against all odds, he has expanded our family, not by falling in love and marrying, but by being accepted into a home pioneered by a Catholic order called the Brothers of Charity, and modeled on the L'Arche living communities.

A Place to Work

I did not know, at the time of our enlightening dinner conversation, back in 1971, that my parents were already actively looking for practical solutions to my brother's future. That same year, five fathers of what we then referred to as "mentally retarded" boys formed a nonprofit company to provide for their son's futures. A few years later, my father joined the organization renamed Decision Enterprises Corporation, or DEC. Its goal was to found workshops that would eventually provide employment for their sons, all of whom were entering their teenage years and would clearly need a great deal of assistance to reach a developmental point where they could hold a job. They opened two training centers, or sheltered workshops, in Montgomery County, Pennsylvania.

I'm not sure what sort of job training was offered in those early years. I do remember my father agonizing over how to create a computer program to teach people like my brother to fry an egg. He seemed to think that anything less complicated than scientific research was an easy task, and that learning how to fry an egg was all one needed to become a short order cook. His program would show a video clip of an egg frying, he thought, and have a button to push at the right time to turn it over. Having never actually fried an egg himself, he thought that knowing when to turn an over-easy egg was all there was to it. I'm not sure how far this misguided project got before it was abandoned. But many other projects succeeded, and the workshops expanded over the years. My brother still works in one of them.

Today, DEC operates five training centers and a variety of other community support services, including independent living and community employment programs. Their vision statement, from their website, is "DEC envisions persons with disabilities living healthy, meaningful, productive and safe lives that are rich in community associations and contributions and who have valued roles in their communities" (www.decmc.org). They supply a good portion of the services to people with intellectual disabilities in Montgomery County.

As my mother predicted, my brother has indeed become a working man. Paul goes to work every weekday from eight to four, at one of the workshops. DEC finds contracts for jobs that cannot be easily automated and are not cost-effective for nondisabled workers. If your company needs six of these and three of those put into a baggie and stapled closed, five hundred times over, Paul's your man. Assuming, of course, that you don't need the baggies until sometime next month. He gets paid based on his production—minimum wage per hour—every time he does as much work as a "normal" person could do in an hour. Some weeks he makes enough money to buy a CD or a DVD.

The place where my brother works is a long, flat concrete building set back from a busy road, behind other utilitarian businesses. There is a long concrete access ramp with sturdy railings next to the concrete stairs. The entryway is a single glass and metal door, which opens on to a beige hallway. A person behind a window next to the door checks for unauthorized visitors. There is a second doorway at the end of the hallway, past a few open office doors. This door is opaque wood, and behind it is a fluorescent-lit room with a concrete floor and cinderblock walls. There are industrial metal shelves along the walls, holding the materials needed for fulfilling the current contracts. There is a small bank of lockers, and a lonely television. The center of the room is filled with tables and chairs, enough to seat maybe fifty workers, or "clients."

This would be a bleak and forbidding place, except for the buzz of excitement coming from those tables. Perhaps this was merely because I arrived at quitting time, but I don't think so. While I was scanning the room for my brother, three different people spotted me and crossed the room to introduce themselves and shake my hand. They were all totally delighted to meet "Paul's sister" and proud to show me the place where they worked.

The clients call their work the "contracts." They also use this word for all the pieces they need to assemble to complete the job, and for the finished product. At the time of my visit, there were two contracts. One was to put a sticker saying "Vote for Senator Greenleaf" on a baggie, then fill it with candy spearmint leaves (which my brother called both "contracts" and "greenleafs").[1] The other was to assemble a paper box and place in it a single ventilator mask and instructions for its use. The boxes were then packed into bigger cardboard boxes to be shipped to the anesthesiologists who will use them. Paul was on the second contract that day, folding flattened paper cut-outs into a small box. He demonstrated for me how it was done. He has developed a worsening tremor in his hands over the years, and it took him a full minute to open the folded paper into a cube and push the tabs at the bottom together to make a box. His face was rapt with effort and concentration, and at the end shone with accomplishment.

I have to mention that, in no financial sense, is this meaningful work. It is boring and trivial and could be done in a few hours by anyone else. The workshop actually loses money on the contracts, and Paul's placement at the workshop is supported by around $1,000 a month of state funds. There are many times when there are no available contracts, and there is no work for the clients to do. During these times, the program is supplemented by music therapy, art therapy, showings of DVDs, and other activities.

In recent years, the sheltered workshop system has come under criticism for creating work that is demeaning and boring, and for causing isolation of the intellectually disabled worker from the mainstream. Many states are phasing them out, in favor of "real" work created in the "real" space and context of money-making businesses (Serres & Howatt, 2015). Indeed, my brother has several friends who are successfully working at such jobs after becoming bored at the workshop. One works at a laundry (with much assistance) and another worked as a greeter and bagger at a grocery store. Paul does not see these possibilities as any better, nor his friends as a degree or so "higher functioning" than he is, though in fact they are.

Paul is seemingly not entirely alone in his view toward work and money. Jamie Berube, the subject of *Life as We Know It* (1996), is the only other adult with intellectual disabilities who has weighed in with a narrative opinion. Jamie has Down syndrome and his father wrote a second book about him at age twenty-six, *Life as Jamie Knows It* (Berube, 2016). Jamie's father states, "Praise for his good work means everything to him; money means almost nothing. *Almost* nothing, because he was definitely very happy with himself to be pulling down two hundred dollars a week . . ." (p. 155). Jamie is "high functioning," a term neither his father

---

[1] This senator is the same person who arranged for meetings to address the issue of aging parents still living with their intellectually disabled sons and daughters, twenty-five years ago. I'm thankful that his support of people with intellectual disabilities has not lost him any elections and that his support continues on a personal as well as political level.

nor I like, but we don't have a better one. In this context it means that Jamie, unlike Paul, understands numbers. Jamie is having trouble finding people who will employ him, but he can earn ten times what my brother does, when he works. It is, of course, still not enough to live on. It is the praise for a job well done, which seemingly is given equally to Paul and Jamie, that is more valuable than the money. Jamie also uses his personal funds to buy music and DVDs.

There is another aspect to working that Jamie, being "higher functioning," is able to convey. Berube writes that Jamie "does not mind the repetitive, sedentary, and intellectually un-stimulating nature of the work. He likes the workplace, and he likes his coworkers. He comes home cheerful every day, happy to be a commuter, happy to be a bit more independent from his parents" (2016, p. 161). Paul, while he is not able to commute on his own, also comes home happy every day, satisfied with his small contribution. Work, as it was for even the severely intellectually disabled people in the L'Arche communities, is not a way to make money, so much as somewhere to go and somewhere to be with other people.

It would I think be quite easy to convince my brother that what he is doing is somehow beneath him. In the name of free choice, a person who was not paying attention to my brother's actual needs could convince him to be dissatisfied with his current work. I hope that no one attempts this. My brother does not need to know that his work is created for his benefit. He does not need to know that his paycheck does not come anywhere near covering his living expenses. He does not even need to know that there are living expenses; this concept is beyond him. He has what he needs and is delighted when he can buy himself a new DVD, with money he made by being a working man.

A Place to Belong

My brother has enjoyed the benefits of several wonderful programs for people with disabilities over the years. His social life in his teens revolved around church activities. I remember vaguely, with some discomfort and embarrassment, attending dances for "mentally retarded" teens at a Presbyterian church. I know that he participated in the Special Olympics for years, mostly as a swimmer. His medals hang from a hook in his room, displayed in a position of prominence. They occupy somewhere around a cubic foot of space. But I was in college when this activity began, and I never attended an event, even when he went to the state championships.

I did witness the work done by the Boy Scouts of America, however. For me, Paul's proudest and most impressive accomplishment came from Troop #254, a troop founded to meet the needs of boys with delayed development. They held their first meetings at the Presbyterian church. My brother joined in 1975. By the next year, all the boys had earned the rank of Scout, which is usually completed in the first month. It was six years before they made it to the next rank, Tenderfoot.

On February 12, 2011, some thirty-five years later, my brother, along with three other members of Troop #254, were invited into the ranks of Eagle Scouts in a crowded ceremony. I decided not to travel halfway across the country to attend. At the time my son was in the Scouts, and working toward Eagle, and I thought it would be boring. Fortunately, a film crew from one of the local TV stations was on hand, so I have a DVD of the whole thing. It was not boring. For Paul, with his never-ending love of any type of reproduction of sound or image, this made the event almost unbearably wonderful. It was also, I believe, a landmark in the history of scouting. There have been other special needs troops, and other handicapped men who have received Eagles, but Troop #254 was one of the first and took the longest. I should have been there.

When they were founded, the members of the troop were all really boys, eleven to fourteen years old. Initially there were somewhere around eight of them, all diagnosed as what was called at the time "trainable" or "educable mentally retarded." Most of the boys had Down syndrome, though my brother and a few others had other diagnoses. Their designation as a Special Needs Troop provided them with appropriate adaptations for all the rank and badge requirements. That included waiving the age maximum to attain Eagle Scout, which is how they came to be able to continue working on it for so long.

There were some rocky times over the years. The fathers all got older, and all but four of the guys had to leave the troop. Some moved away, but many dropped out when their parents were unable to take them to meetings any more. But four of them persisted in attending meetings every Thursday night. They were all both too old and too young to be Eagle Scouts. Measured in years, they were all much too old. Scouts without handicaps must fulfill the multitude of requirements and service projects before the age of eighteen. Some don't finish in time and became ineligible for the rank. Measured by the old scale of "mental age" none of the guys were developmentally much past age ten. Almost every requirement had to be adapted so that they could do it. It required a lot of work and a lot of persistence and a lot of support.

I assume, for example, that the troop got some major adaptations on the requirements for the First Aid Merit Badge. The badge requires a fairly thorough understanding of what to do in basic medical emergencies. My son had to learn CPR. Though Paul is absolutely thrilled by medical emergencies, including when they happen to himself, his understanding of medical care comes down to, "D-5 double-you, STAT!" He learned this from watching his favorite show *Emergency!* when it was on UHS TV in reruns every night forever. He's also pretty good at shouting "Call 9-1-1!" in a very loud, demanding voice, accompanied by an exaggerated frown, and unfortunately not always reserved for actual emergencies. This was pretty cute when he was eleven or so, but somewhat disconcerting in a middle-aged man.

Many things that Troop #254 has done were ever so much harder for them than for other troops. They went, for example, on all the required camping trips, including a "wilderness" trip, with no tents or cooking gear. It rained the whole weekend. Try that with four nondisabled middle-aged guys and see how far you get. My brother walks by essentially falling forward, catching himself just in time with each step, which means he needs assistance on anything other than a flat surface. I can only imagine camping with four men whose balance is poor and will take twenty minutes to go to the bathroom when it isn't 200 yards away down a path through the woods. And yet, they did all that was required: camping, cooking over an open fire, hiking, and swimming.

They completed their Eagle projects, one of the last and most difficult requirements. And it was clearly as worthy and successful as any other Eagle project I've heard about. They all did the same project, which was to collect food for a local charity. But they did it individually, each at a different church. They set up a collection date, then handed out flyers and made a speech about their project at a Sunday service. They helped each other carry the donations to the food shelf. I suspect that they got boatloads of food, rather more than would have been procured by any other Boy Scouts. I'm sure those speeches, in halting, deep voices, were heart-rending.

Did they have help? Of course. But so did every other Eagle Scout. I've been told that no one becomes an Eagle Scout without a certain amount of effort from their families. As far as I can tell, soliciting help is an integral and necessary part of all Eagle projects. I believe that no other scouts in the history of scouting have worked so hard or so long or so persistently to become Eagle Scouts. Nor has anyone worked against such enormous odds. There is no reasonable way that any of these guys could have earned this honor. So, against all reason, they continued chipping away at this, one requirement at a time, step by tiny step, every Thursday night for thirty-five years.

I cannot claim that becoming an Eagle Scout in any way justifies or increases the value of my brother's life. From a purely utilitarian standpoint, my brother's life has a negative value. Growing up, he took more than his fair share of medical and educational resources. If I want to be uncharitable, I can complain that he took more than his fair share of my family's resources, including some that should have been mine. At this point, between maintaining the home where he lives and the sheltered workshop where he spends his days, he costs somewhere around $50,000 per year of taxpayer money. We, as a capitalist society, get nothing back from that. He does not, in fact, even earn his tiny paycheck.

To see value, we must create a new definition for it, disassociated from economics altogether. Yet, despite centuries of philosophical thinking, we do not have another scale that measures the worth of lives. We have no idea what one person must accomplish before the debt incurred by life can be justified. I suspect that all of us fall short in the balance.

Can I claim that my brother is our teacher, by persevering all those years? No. Can I claim that he is special, some sort of sainted example? Not at all. My brother is not a saint nor does he have anything special to offer to humanity. Paul is merely himself, a person whose needs are so obvious that even the least observant of us cannot fail to notice them. It is the people who attended to and met those needs over the years who have something to teach us. Ian Brown writes of his son Walker, "The face of God? Sorry, no. Walker is more like a mirror, reflecting much back, my choices included" (2011, p. 286). Those who spent time looking at the reflection of their choices understand the value of care.

There were almost 150 Eagle Scouts at the ceremony, spanning all ages from teenagers to middle-aged men. Troop #254, it turns out, involved many people, including a scoutmaster who, not only devoted years to the troop, but linked with other troops as well. Over the years, a succession of young men came from other troops to help out. A small crowd of them came to the ceremony to celebrate their mutual accomplishment. By their attendance, the village that made four fifty-year-old intellectually disabled men into Eagle Scouts made a clear statement of the value of that achievement in their own lives.

Two years later, both of my brothers traveled halfway across the country to attend my son's Eagle ceremony. The last thing in that ceremony was a recitation of the Eagle Scout Oath, by all the Eagle Scouts in attendance. There were nowhere near 150 of them. But my brother stood with the others, unsteadily, in his Eagle-decorated uniform, while they recited the Oath. Even repeating five words at a time, Paul had trouble keeping up, his blurry words lagging into the silence after everyone else had finished each phrase. No one could mistake that he had spent decades carefully learning to say those words in that order. No one could mistake how difficult that had been. Nor could they mistake his enormous pride in being able to say them. His smile and his enthusiasm were unflagging, a reminder that this ceremony, and all of their accomplishments, was no small thing.

Michael Berube writes, "The world is a better place for his [Jamie's] being in it, I am quite sure of that, but the most important metric is his enjoyment of the world, not the world's enjoyment of him" (2016, p. 189). Paul's enjoyment of scouting was part of his place in the world, and, by this "most important" metric, that enjoyment is the value of his life.

In the end, there is perhaps nothing that anyone can do that will absolutely prove the value of anyone's life. But enjoyment, as well as pride and enthusiasm, is cyclical. It is nearly impossible to witness Paul's pride, enthusiasm, and enjoyment without responding to it in kind. If his caregivers contributed to Paul's enjoyment, they also created enjoyment for themselves. Perhaps the best that anyone can hope for is to have a small effect on the lives of some people beyond those of one's immediate family. Against all odds, Paul has joined the community of humanity, touching the lives of strangers, and perhaps making them a tiny bit better.

A Place to Call Home

The history of out-of-home placement for children with intellectual disabilities is full of stories of unfortunate experiences. The behavioral conditioning used to treat Noah Greenfeld's autism at one residential facility left bruises (Greenfeld, 1986). Sumner Hart, a fifty-year-old with autism who had lived with his mother his whole life, smeared himself with feces and then ran away from a mental hospital in California (Hart, 1989). Stories of unethical experiments done at the Willowbrook State School in New York, the Fernald School in Massachusetts, and others, are widespread. Images of the poor conditions at Pennhurst, an institution in eastern Pennsylvania, were documented in a five-part television series shown in 1968. Pennhurst, falling into ruins after its closure in 1987, was reopened for Halloween in 2010 as a gory haunted house and attracted long lines despite controversy and the $50 admission price (Tarabay, 2010). This ensures that its memory will be, not only preserved, but also exaggerated.

However, institutional care was not always untenable. There are other stories with happier endings. As long ago as 1940, successful writer Pearl S. Buck placed her daughter Carol at the Training School in Vineland, New Jersey. Carol had PKU, a metabolic disease which results in slow developmental regression throughout childhood, whose cause had not yet been discovered. Carol was then nine years old and had spent most of the previous year under her mother's tutelage, frustrated at her inability to learn to read (Buck, 1950). At the training school, she learned the things she needed to know: self-care, table manners, and to verbalize her needs. She listened to music on her radio and participated in the Special Olympics. She lived there happily until her death in 1992 (Christ & Finger, 2004).

Ted Hart, Sumner's nephew, who, like his uncle, had fairly severe autism, did well in the group home where he had been placed at age eleven. Ian Brown's son Walker also became too much to handle at home by age eleven and was placed in a group home. At the time of the publication of his father's memoir, Walker was still there and seemed to be thriving. He shared a room, with pictures of his family on the walls, with two other nonverbal, intellectually disabled boys who perhaps were becoming friends. After frequent visits home, he seemed happy to return, though, of course, Walker had no way of expressing that verbally.

The decision to place their children elsewhere was not made easily. Both fathers spend many pages justifying their decision, as well as dealing with real grief at the loss of the presence of their son. Ted Hart's father stresses the toll that caregiving had taken on the rest of his family and the growing impossibility of meeting Ted's needs, then states, "Placing Ted out of our home merely for the comfort of the rest of us seemed unforgivably wrong and immoral. How could we live with our consciences if we sacrificed the weakest, most vulnerable member of our family for the convenience of those of us who had more natural gifts?" (1989, p. 184). Walker's father, no longer able to meet Walker's twenty-four-hour needs, wrestles also with the guilt of failure, "Who wants to admit you've had a child and can't raise him? (Brown, 2011, p. 108).

Research based on interviews with nine mothers of children with autism regarding their decision to place their children outside their home, suggests that Brown and Hart are not alone in either the guilt they felt or how they dealt with it. The mothers in the study had placed their children in group homes at an average age of eleven years old, just as for Ted and Walker. The mothers demonstrated understanding that placing a child with a disability outside the home is now unusual and that sending a child away is not consistent with current ideals of proper mothering. Thus, they felt that placement was viewed as culturally and morally unacceptable, and as a "deviation from the norm." They expressed feelings of guilt, inadequacy, and stigmatization. Some also expressed grief at the loss of the child's presence in their home; one of the mothers called her decision "a near death experience" (Corman, 2013, p. 1325).

However, several years after placement, most of the mothers reported their decision as unavoidable, mostly because their child's behavior had become uncontrollable and dangerous. They still felt guilty but were willing to blame a lack of social supports such as respite care and day programs for failing to help their child. They also were able to transfer some of the guilt they felt to the condition of autism, the cause of their child's behavior problems. The researcher recommended that the definition of good mothering should be extended to include families of children with disabilities that must live outside their parents' home, a point with which I absolutely agree (Corman, 2013). That this suggestion is needed at all attests to the moral distress that parents must work through in this situation.

There are a few narrative indications that living outside the home has some benefits for the child as well as for his overworked family. Both Ted and Walker seemed to thrive in their new homes. Ted's father reported that his new group home "offer[ed] Ted more advantages than the family home" (Hart, 1989, p. 184), including a stable and predictable schedule, and round-the-clock support. There is a scene toward the end of the book in which Ted's caregivers and social workers sit down with his parents to discuss a recent deterioration in behavior. Together, in a good example of responsiveness, they figure out what Ted is trying to tell them through his nonverbal cues and initiate a successful plan to respond to it. Ian Brown noted that his son became a different and perhaps happier person in his new environment. After Walker had spent some time in the group home, Brown observes, "But it's [Walker's] emotional confidence that's leaping forward. Living only in our world, I'm sure, he saw his limitations everywhere. In his new vacation home, as I think of it, surrounded by peers, he's as solid as anyone. I hope that is the gift we gave him by giving him up" (2011, p. 109).

Placement outside the home is perhaps a rare necessity and not the first choice of any parent. But for many families, like those of Ted and Walker, caregiving in a family setting is not a viable or sustainable option. The decision to place a child during the teenage years should not be framed as a failure of caregiving and parenting ability. It is a source of guilt and grief that are, perhaps, dealt with by blaming the uncontrollable nature of the disability. But it is also assuaged by the possibility that the child might thrive in the new environment. Once it became clear that Walker was doing well in his group home, Brown was even able to frame his choice as a gift he had given his son. He says, of Walker, "He is becoming a different boy there, in his other house. He has a life of his own, something I thought he'd never experience" (p. 247). He has, in fact, given his son a chance, not just at a tiny fraction of independence, but to develop in ways that are different from what he would have experienced at home, influenced by a different set of caregivers.

Parents who place their adult children outside the home are subject to the same guilt and stigma. Though we expect typical kids to move out at some point, and in fact make jokes about people who fail to do so, many expect parents to continue to care for adult children if they cannot achieve independence. Yet there is a long wait list for placements, and a fear that no place is better than the family home. When my family was touring group homes in several states, looking for a place for my brother, we were warned about the possibility of callous treatment, staff indifference, and even theft. High staff turnover and low pay were the presumed causes of this, a problem which is no different today. The combination of societal expectations and lack of trust in available placements, along with a never-ending wait list, contributed to my parents' paralysis at finding a new home for my brother. A place did not arrive until several years after my father's first heart attack.

We assume, perhaps on very little evidence, that moving out is both beneficial and necessary for the development of a typical child. Why should it not be just as true for a child with a disability? Leaving aside the issue of whether parents benefit from release from their caregiving duties, it is possible that moving out might be beneficial for the child. Many people, including the founder of L'Arche communities, Jean Vanier, believe that even people with severe intellectual disabilities deserve a place of their own, apart from their families and parents (Brown, 2011, p. 196). Parents who have done the task of extreme caregiving following tenets of attentiveness and responsiveness have provided an environment in which a child can thrive. But remaining perpetually at home might restrict the opportunity for others to contribute to the now-adult person's self-expression. There may well be advantages to moving out, as long as equally responsive caregivers can be found.

There is some evidence that living with parents, at least in adulthood, may not always be the best circumstance for intellectually disabled adults.

Researchers have pointed out that while adults with intellectual disabilities appear content and seem to prefer to remain with family members, clearly their future becomes more uncertain as their parents age (Weeks et al., 2009). A review of the literature on intellectually disabled people living at home documented that the home provided strong family relationships, the possibility of the intellectually disabled person supplying support to an aging parent, and more stable behavior. But it also found that those who still lived with parents or family had many unmet service needs, more use of neuroleptic medications, were more overweight (in Down syndrome), and had a smaller network of friends. Adults living with their parents often reported no friends that were not also friends with a parent (Seltzer & Krauss, 2001). Another study, a survey of 852 people with intellectual disabilities over the age of nineteen, found that those who were living with their parents had less access to necessary supports, including help with activities of daily living and crisis intervention. They also had less opportunity to develop community connections and were less likely to participate in community activities than those living in group homes (Stainton et al., 2011).

These studies rely largely on parents and support workers to answer the questions on written questionnaires. Those few that interviewed people with intellectual disabilities directly were limited to fairly high-functioning individuals. The studies based on interviews don't necessarily agree with those based on questionnaires. In interviews, several (fifteen) intellectually disabled adults reported they prefer to live "in close proximity to their peers and in large groups in the community rather than in small, dispersed community housing" (Shaw et al., 2011, p. 895). However, in a different study, parents reported a high preference for having their intellectually disabled child living in a small, supervised home with fewer than four residents (Weeks et al., 2009).

My brother cannot give you his opinion on this matter. Or, rather, my brother could be talked into giving you any opinion you wished him to express. None of the research papers quite captures this naïve pliability, though I am sure my brother is not unique in this regard. His worldview does not include things outside his experiences, and he cannot speculate on the way things could be different for him. Nor does he have an understanding of why you might wish to hear one answer over another. Mostly, he wants to agree with you, unless you touch on a negative past experience. Nonetheless, he has, without even realizing it, won the wait list lottery with one of the best placements available. In the wake of my parents' activism, Paul was offered a spot at a new sort of group home, being pioneered by the Brothers of Charity, a worldwide Catholic Order headquartered in Philadelphia. I cannot imagine a situation in which he could be more content.

The house where my brother lives now is a lovely brick building, probably best described as a manor house, located in a quiet suburb not too far from the Pennsylvania Turnpike. It sits on an immaculate, tree-studded lawn, or, perhaps, estate. At the end of a sweeping driveway, there is a small parking lot bounded by a low stone wall. The asphalt comes right up to the front door, which is usually open and lined with plants and welcome signs.

Inside there is an atrium decorated with antique furniture and religious paintings. Straight ahead there is, visible through an open double doorway, a dark wood table that is obviously an altar. There is almost always an enormous array of fresh flowers beside it. To the right are offices and a gracious receiving room, which is rarely in use. All the action is to the left, where an industrial-sized kitchen gives way to the communal dining room. That leads to the common sitting room and the hallway with four college-dorm-sized rooms and one shared bathroom. There is an exercise room, four more dorm rooms, and another bathroom downstairs. My brother's room is the second one from the end, upstairs.

The inhabitants of the house, named Triest Hall, include four Brothers, who live and work there, and eight intellectually disabled men. The sister of one of the Brothers comes in to help with the cooking. They all go to work in the mornings, the Brothers to the Church offices, and the guys to their various workshops and adapted community jobs. At home, they enjoy public and private time, and know each other's favorite activities. They live together, cook and eat together, and do chores together. They do favors for each other, and play jokes on each other as well.

When we were in college, my siblings started referring to each other by our relationships. Paul took up this eagerly and has since then called me Sister Lisa and his brother, Brother Walter. So he saw nothing unusual in adopting Brother Mike and Brother John and Brother Denis and Brother Anton into his family. The families of the other residents at Triest Hall often ask after this mysterious, invisible "Brother Walter" who Paul is always talking about. My brother Paul is the most impaired of the guys, and no one else has misunderstood the nature of their relationship. But Paul is correct. In many ways, he has found four new brothers. And so have I.

According to Brother John, the other residents are referred to by the county as their "clients," but everyone at the house calls them simply "the guys." The home is supervised by the Montgomery County Department of Developmental Disabilities and Behavioral Health (MCDDDBH), which administers and supervises all the residential programs in the county. According to his most recent Individual Service Plan (ISP), the county pays $40,739.46 per year for my brother's care. This comes from state funds and from money paid to my brother via Social Security. (The home is not eligible for federal money because the federal waivers that pay for housing through the Americans with Disabilities Act are only good for situations where four or fewer disabled people are housed.) Because the Brothers of Charity perform their caregiving work without pay, Triest Hall is actually much cheaper for the state than most other homes.

There is no official wait list for living at Triest Hall, though the Brothers are sometimes approached by families seeking placement for their son. The wait list for residential placement is maintained by MCDDDBH, who will refer new clients if a position becomes available. They, appropriately, take only men. They prefer older men with mild to moderate intellectual disabilities, whose parents are aging. They cannot take a client with violent behavior nor can they take someone who is unable to handle the stairs. My brother was one of the first eight guys. In the twenty-five years he has lived there, only five new clients have been accepted. Two of those were to replace original residents whose needs were not being adequately met. The other three vacancies were due to deaths from complications of aging.

Nor is there much turnover in the staff. Brother Mike retired, but he still lives at Triest Hall. Brothers occasionally arrive, often from other countries, to observe the community and to do their own mission work. Several have returned to their home countries to start their own homes for intellectually disabled people. Brother Anton will soon be returning to the Philippines, where the Brothers of Charity have two institutions for children with disabilities. Eventually, I imagine, someone new will arrive. Triest Hall has become the model for a successful home, and there are now about a dozen homes like it around the world.

There is no requirement for religious affiliation. Half the current residents are Jewish. The guys are encouraged to spend holidays with their families, but this has become less possible over the years as the parents of residents have aged and siblings have moved away. All holidays are acknowledged and celebrated. Last year the Brothers held a Seder for those residents who couldn't get home for Passover. They used a service they found on the internet, and one of the Jewish men recited the prayer for Chanukah, since that is the only one he had been able to memorize. And all the residents are invited to attend the daily evening prayer service in the chapel room. Another Jewish resident never misses one.

When I asked Brother John about their philosophy of care, he gave me a book about Jean Vanier and L'Arche. The Brothers of Charity have embraced the L'Arche philosophy of "living with" the mentally disabled. They also believe in holding an attitude of "gentle teaching" that is based on "solidarity" with the mentally disabled. This solidarity requires mutual respect and reciprocal acceptance, and recognizes the humanity in everyone (Terruwe & Kroft, 2006, p. 21). Because of this, the Brothers' relationships with my brother have changed from that of a stranger, about whom they knew nothing except what my parents told them, to people who know him well. They know his concerns, his quirks, and his needs. Brother John shrugs and says, "We've lived together for twenty-five years," as though no other way is possible. Their relationships with the other guys have developed similarly, from people they learned about through their families or the county's ISP to someone they know well. And their care and concern is reciprocated.

Brother John says that he did not expect to get anything out of this arrangement but has learned things that he never expected. He does not quite express Vanier's impression that the intellectually disabled are holy. But he thinks "the guys" might have special abilities in the "emotional and psychological" arena. He has admired their level of patience, their unconditional trust, their lack of resentment, and their willingness to establish a relationship.

I believe, as I have said previously, that it is in the caregiving itself that this learning occurs. One must be open to it. One must be willing to listen to those slow, deep voices, which say sometimes seemingly outrageous things. It is often necessary to ask for several repetitions to understand. It requires patience, calmness, and a certain amount of creativity. And from such gentleness, comes mutual respect, if not love, and mutual growth. I could tell several stories about how my brother has continued to mature in his new home. Many of these are ways which would not have been possible if he had stayed with my parents. Like Walker, he has become someone new at his new home. I will restrict myself to one of the most recent examples.

We all grow, whether we wish to or not, after the death of a parent. My father died when Paul was forty-six and had been living with the Brothers for twenty years. His death was not unexpected, and we were all worried about how Paul would deal with the event. Paul carries emotional upsets with him, unabated, often for decades. Any reminder of past problems, illnesses, or deaths (including one of the deaths at Triest Hall) will trigger an emotional response unchanged from when the event first happened.

However, Paul's best friend Huey died in hospice at Triest Hall, of early dementia associated with Down syndrome, a year before my father's death. Paul had been at his bedside and faced the death under the gentle teaching of his Brothers. It seemed that Paul had benefited emotionally from his inclusion in Huey's death and funeral. And so, my family had two funerals for my father. One was a standard affair at a funeral home near the community where Dad spent most of his retirement. The other was a few months later at Triest Hall. Paul came to both of them.

The first funeral was attended by about one hundred people, mostly college-professor friends of my sister and a scattering of people from the retirement community. There were the usual stately rows of chairs, facing a small urn surrounded by photographs and flowers. There was a pastor from my sister's church. In the middle of the service, Paul began to cry. Now, crying is something Paul does with his whole being, and it is not quiet. Perhaps a better description would be that he began to wail in huge, wet sobs. Heads turned, some in sympathy and some in alarm. One of the heads was my mother's. She motioned to me frantically, embarrassed, asking me to take him away. I knew this because I had agreed to it in advance. We had all heard Paul cry before.

And so, I took my brother's hand and led him, still sobbing, from the room. On the way down the aisle, I decided that the timing of his tears was totally correct. We sat together on a couch in a different room, near a box of tissues, and both cried until we were done. Paul turns out to be a very good person to cry with. His grief was uncomplicated and undemanding, needing only to be shared until it ran itself out.

The second funeral was a Catholic service held in the chapel in Triest Hall. There were very few people there, just the Brothers, and the guys, and my family. Some of the Boy Scouts came too. The service was presided over by someone with the title of Reverend Monsignor and was quite formal. Paul sat behind me with Brother John and, of course, in the middle of the service, began to cry. My mother turned to me with the same horrified, embarrassed look, but Brother John raised a restraining hand and gently shook his head. One of the guys quietly moved to sit on Paul's other side and leaned a little bit toward him. The Monsignor did not even seem to notice. Supported on both sides by people who were not embarrassed by his disability, Paul's sobbing abated in just a few minutes.

My mother's reasons for having me remove Paul from the first service are complicated and include a desire to prevent him from being hurt by the attention of people who do not know him. It also includes a desire to prevent others from being made uncomfortable by him. The first service was for her, and it was fine to remove Paul from it, but the second was almost entirely for him, and he needed to stay. He did not need to be protected from an embarrassment he did not notice or care about. He needed to share in our ceremonial expression of grief.

He seems to found comfort in it. He has none of the lack of understanding, anger, and inexpressible pain that we were dreading. He does sometimes tell others about it. He puts on his enormous frown and blurts out, "Paul Freitag's father . . . DIED." (He always uses his full name and third person for this. We don't know why.) When he says it to me, I just say, "Yes, I know, he was my father too," and we both are sad for a bit. When he tells a total stranger, we explain, and allow that person to express condolences as well. His unhappiness does not last long, as is appropriate for a grief now several years old.

The Brothers know who Paul is. They know his quirks and faults, along with his strengths. They live and eat with him. They are not embarrassed by him. They know how far, and when, he can be nudged ever so slightly toward personal growth. And even though there are many childish things that Paul can't do, they have guided him to a mature understanding of life and death.

It is obvious that there is much that we do not know about how to create the best living situations for a person with intellectual disabilities who cannot live independently. We all agree that respect and as much independence as possible are essential. However, it also should be obvious that, while common needs can be catalogued and sometimes even measured, each person and family has a different set of needs. Each living situation is also different.

A variety of placement situations have emerged in the decades since my parents helped close the institutions. These vary from a single individual living with some support from family or a paid care worker, to larger homes where many people are cared for by workers on shifts. A review of recent progress in housing for adults with intellectual disabilities concluded that there was no one particular way that could be clearly demonstrated to be the best. The single determinant of successful outcome for the residents was the way staff provided the needed support (Mansell, 2006). Yet there is no agreement as to how staff could or should be trained to be supportive. I have two simple suggestions based on my brother's life with the Brothers and the philosophy of L'Arche: eating together and quiet listening.

We will not find very many people who are willing, like the Brothers of Charity or Jean Vanier, to take religious vows or dedicate their lives to care. We cannot expect many people to give up their current lives to "live with" the tens of thousands of people with intellectual disabilities who are currently on wait lists for placement. But I think it would be possible to bring the idea of sharing meals into many of our currently existing living situations. When the staff of, say, a nursing home, retreats into a hidden room to have lonely meals in shifts, that sends a message to both care workers and residents about their respective value. Everyone loses a chance for meaningful interaction. Breaking bread together is a human ritual, expressing respect, community, and mutual service.

Eating with my brother is no more socially awkward than eating with anyone else; it doesn't even take longer. He methodically works his way around his plate, eating all of one thing before proceeding to the next. At the end, he gulps whatever drink is available in one, long swallow. This can be alarming, but he hasn't yet run out of breath. He has only once interrupted a meal by a pronouncement about going to college that shook my worldview. And while he hasn't really learned to take turns in conversation, it is possible to talk quite a lot while he is eating.

Listening to my brother is perhaps more important than eating with him. Your worldview won't perhaps be altered by listening patiently, once again, to that thing about movie projectors. Listening to my brother is frustrating, time-consuming, and, often, boring. His words are slow, slurred, and difficult to understand. He has a tendency to repeat himself endlessly. It is very tempting to cut him off after a few words, supplying your own interpretation. But it is the act of listening, not the information being recited, that is important. If you work at understanding him, staying open to discovering his meaning, his concerns, and his needs, you might discover in yourself patience, charity, and the ability to slow down.

Listening is not currently on the official list of the things my brother requires. His ISP is a well-meant and considered list of the services that he can be documented to need, and which must be provided by right. It is an example of the current attitude toward caring for him, as is the preferred word for referring to him at both workshop and government-provided home: client. As Brother John says, "In the County ISP, the person is defined as an object of need to which services are provided." But if you spend any time listening quietly to my brother, you learn that he is more than a summary of his many needs. Reading his ISP, you learn about his disability. Listening to him, you discover his humanity and, possibly, your own.

Listening must be done on an individual, rather than an institutional, level. It requires a small attitudinal shift, from one of service to one of openness to needs. Jean Vanier also found that, as he lived with people with intellectual disabilities, his attitude shifted from "wanting to do things for" toward "listening to." According to one biographer, his ability to do this was "a revolution which was no doubt made possible by his own openness and readiness to be shaped by experience and events" (Spink, 1991, p. 42). This openness and readiness to learn seems to me a good description of responsiveness. Attentive and open listening to both verbal and nonverbal clues allow for care based upon who the person is, rather than what the current theory states that they need. And responding to (or being shaped by) what is learned, rather than relying on one's preconceived notions, is not only a way of discovering unrevealed needs, but also a way of discovering the person who has them.

And so we see that the primary determinant of my brother's future has been that people in his life are following the moral precepts of Tronto's phases of care. He is surrounded by people both at home and at work who are both attentive to his needs and taking the responsibility for providing them. His caregivers are beyond competent in their abilities. But it is the closing of that cycle of care that is the most important. The things he has to say, limited and perhaps boring as they may be, are listened to by people to whom those needs, feelings, and expressions are important. He responds with all the love and joy, and dismay and sorrow, as the rest of us.

We still have much to learn from the caregivers who are willing to listen to him.

CHAPTER 9 | Conclusion
Caring With

NO ONE HAS ever doubted that raising a child with special needs is an enormous task. There are some who might feel that it is not very different from raising a "typical" child, but, while there are many things in common, I maintain that the sum of the tasks involved is more complex. The physical, financial, and emotional toll is higher. The tasks can be arduous, isolating, and misunderstood. That is why I have called it extreme caregiving.

This does not mean that the work is completely without rewards. This does not mean that it must be more heartbreaking, though it can be. It certainly does not mean that it is not well worth doing. Nor does it mean that we should somehow prevent the burden of caregiving by preventing the existence of the child. It just means that it is more work.

This book has attempted to bring that work into the open by categorizing and describing it using the phases of care proposed by Joan Tronto (1993). I have done my best to listen to academics in the fields of medicine, nursing, bioethics, and disability studies, but my main source of information has been published biographical material from the parents who are doing extreme caregiving. I have also brought my personal experiences into the analysis.

In the first two of Tronto's phases of care, we have seen that extreme caregiving parents are called to a high level of attentiveness toward their children and must take on responsibilities that are both unexpected and outside the experience of many parents. They must learn to attend to monitors and medications, multiple appointments and insurance claims. In addition to becoming parents, they must become care coordinators and educators and medical caregivers. On top of that, they often must also become advocates, defending their child's right to a place in the world.

And this must often be done against a backdrop of uncertainty about the child's medical condition and future.

In the third phase of care, competent caregiving, many extreme caregiving parents attain a high level of medical knowledge, mostly unsupported and unacknowledged by medical professionals. The search for information that will help their child becomes, for some, a lifelong quest. Yet despite their success in learning, and their finely honed ability to coordinate all the parts of their child's care, they rarely claim any expertise. In fact, they seem more likely to describe themselves as failures, negating or hiding the high degree of competence they have achieved.

Caregivers in the fourth phase of care, care-receiving, are called upon to elicit a response to care from their charges regarding the appropriateness and effectiveness of the care that has been given. Since children can neither describe the care they require nor, at least initially, coherently verbalize a response, this phase is somewhat different for all parents. To determine the child's needs, parents must remain open to the nonverbal cues that pass back and forth during the process of giving care. These cues are often incomprehensible to those not actively involved with the child. The nonverbal child is thus dependent on the parents, not only for bodily care, but also for interpreting these cues for the outside world. For extreme caregiving parents, this often means developing an exquisite sensitivity to signs of illness or discomfort in an infant with extra needs, as well as translating those needs for medical providers.

Since Tronto's theories include a virtue-based ethic of care, I have also begun to analyze the moral qualities and implications of the work of extreme caregiving. Taking on new responsibilities is moral as well as physical work. The moral effort involved in living with uncertainty, sorting through conflicting emotions, and unexpectedly choosing to perform new tasks should not be underestimated.

Perhaps the most difficult moral task for the parent, however, is the holding of the child's identity, particularly if there is intellectual delay. As the child responds to care, the parents begin to assemble a personality from nonverbal cues. In interpreting the child's needs, the parents inevitably form an idea of the child's personality and begin constructing an identity and story for the child. The child who remains minimally verbal or nonverbal is reliant on the parents' interpretations for an extended period of time. For some of these children, the story their parents create about them is the only life narrative that the child will have. The construction of identity that this entails is an immense moral responsibility.

The recognition of the work that comes with extreme caregiving has been obstructed by the same societal barriers that have served to make all care work invisible. Caregiving is rarely recognized for the necessary and important work that it is. In both politics and in many forms of ethics, the need for care is a barely acknowledged problem, to be dealt with by individuals in isolation and silence. As a result, care is done largely by the least advantaged people, and care work is both underpaid and unappreciated.

The work of caregiving is not only invisible, but we have also seen that many parents feel they must hide the difficulties they might be having, maintaining a cheerful and optimistic attitude lest they be seen as failing to cope. Within the medical system, a parent who admits to difficulties can be rewarded, not with help, but by being labeled as incompetent or uncaring. We have seen that some parents fear this as grounds for removal of the child from the parent's care. Outside of medicine—particularly in the educational and political arenas—parents are constantly called upon to defend their child's needs and advocate for their rights to any services received. Even a simple trip outside the home can result in a challenge, as strangers react unpredictably to the presence of a child with disabilities.

Ian Brown asks a question for all parents who are extreme caregivers. He has been contemplating the nature of art and is looking for some value to his son's life, not because he personally doubts his value, but because others seem to need such justification. He is also desperately tired, and hopes that if he can persuade anyone else of his son's value, they will offer aid. He writes,

> Walker has the same effect as the ballet: they both can reveal the larger shape of the world. He is one of the pools where hope resides.
>
> So to anyone who wonders about the potential value of a severely disabled child, and the possible meaning of a penumbral life passed mostly in pain, that's one possibility. What if Walker's life is a work of art in progress—possibly a collective work of art? Would that persuade you to take care of him for me? (2011, p. 243)

Whether we choose to recognize Walker's value as a work of art, his need is undeniable. The meeting of that immense need has been assigned solely to his family. What would, in fact, persuade us to help Brown, and other parents like him, to take care of their children? And how might we go about doing it?

I have said that I do not believe that help for people like Brown and his son will be found within the current thrust of medicine and medical research, which is dedicated to discovering cures and eliminating risk factors. Medical advances cannot be expected to provide immediate cures for all forms of disability. But, too often, while we are waiting for those scientific miracles, no one is paying particular attention to the needs of those children who are presumed to be hoping for that cure.

In addition, no matter how rigorous we are in screening and prevention, we will not be able to eliminate all forms of disability. Nor does screening provide relief for the hundreds of thousands of children with disabilities who already exist. So far, the push for screening has resulted in a fair amount of blame being placed on the parents of children with special needs, who can be treated as though it is proper for them to suffer the consequences of a decision that they very often did not even make.

Instead, more work must be done to ease the lives of children with disabilities by accommodating their needs in the home, at school, and in society. Michael Berube, the parent of a man with Down syndrome, also recommends putting aside hopes for cures and instead concentrating on aid. His son would benefit immeasurably from a slightly restructured world that could better accommodate his needs. He writes, "the discourse of the cure is everywhere, and the discourse of the reasonable accommodation, so far as I can see, is understood only by those people who already know something about disability" (2016, p. 89). It is possible that some of the money currently spent on biomedical research might be more effectively spent on accommodations for existing disabilities, which would immediately be rendered less disabling.

In addition to funding medical research, I believe that caregiving itself should be funded, both in the form of direct aid to relieve the burden of care and in the form of research to discover what parents are doing that is most effective. In fact, caregiving might even be considered as a reasonable "cure" for many disabling conditions. Consider the vast success of keeping children with intellectual disabilities at home rather than hiding them in institutions. Attentive, competent, and responsive caregiving has resulted in leaps of intellectual ability in children with Down syndrome, for example, and has by itself had better results than any enhancing medication or single therapy developed in the past half-century.

Yet this still leaves the enormous physical and moral task that is extreme caregiving to be done by parents largely in isolation. I have said that part of the responsibility for care falls on the medical system, which seems much more eager to save the lives of children than to assist in the day-to-day realities of their care. Some researchers agree that medical providers and support staff must assume a larger part to support caregiving.

One of the efforts to support parents comes from the movement for perinatal hospice. This is an emerging program to provide support for women who do not wish to abort a fetus diagnosed by prenatal testing with a potentially fatal condition. The programs include prenatal care for the mother and psychosocial support for the family. They also include support once the child is born. In a paper promoting perinatal hospice, philosopher Aaron Cobb, reports, "The parents who have received a diagnosis that their child has a significantly life-limiting condition often lack the capacities and resources essential to care for their child. Physicians, nurses, counselors, social workers, neighbors, friends, and extended family can seek to tend to needs of the parents and their unborn children" (2016, p. 31). Perhaps that team is sufficient to provide needed caregiving aid for the parents, assuming, of course, that the mother's health insurance covers it. However, generally, the infants born with conditions that qualify for perinatal hospice will live at most a few months.

We have seen that many infants live longer than a few months. Ronan Rapp, who had Tay-Sachs disease, a fatal condition, lived for two years. And Samuel, whose prenatal assessment of Cornelia DeLange syndrome included several potentially life-limiting problems, was still doing well at age eleven. We have seen that over years of extreme care, friends and even relatives fall away, daunted by the persistent health crises and complexity of care. And that, while the medical system does offer ongoing support, the multiple required appointments and interactions come with their own burdens.

I do not believe that support from the medical community, even if increased from the current level will be enough. Cobb goes on to say that parents who face a diagnosis of a life-limiting condition need "a community that enables the parent to see that their activities manifest important goods, goods essential to a well-lived human life. It is a community that helps the parent to see that their love is neither futile nor wasted. It is a community that affirms the value and gifted quality of the child's life" (2016, p. 35). I believe that such a community is necessary to support any parents of any child with special needs, not just those with potentially fatal conditions. More importantly, however, I believe that the community support must extend beyond emotional affirmation to the provision of actual hands-on help with caregiving.

In her recent book, *Caring Democracy*, Joan Tronto (2013) has proposed a fifth phase of care, which she calls "caring with." This is the phase in which we as a society become attentive to the need for care, take responsibility for the work that has to be done, adequately care for both the person in need of care and the people providing that care, and listen to their report of their needs. She maintains that this can be done within a democratic society by changing the way we think about dependency.

At this point, our society and our democracy are based on an ideal of autonomy and personal choice that has no room for dependency. Our social policies, financial system, and even much of our philosophical thinking tend to ignore that dependency is a fact of life; all of us required care as children and very likely will be dependent on others again in illness or old age. This lack of acknowledgment has led to the idea that a need for care is aberrant, an unlikely annoyance that we must all deal with on our own. Tronto (2013) proposes that we bring caring to the front of our public process by becoming a democracy that "cares with." She wishes to put the recognition and fulfilling of needs at the center of our decision-making process. Rather than promoting financial success and autonomous isolation, a caring democracy will place its pride in the successful meeting of needs. Once we have equal access to care, and the assurance that our own needs will be met, we become free to care for others. Now that we have catalogued and begun to recognize the caregiving work being done, the need for change is obvious.

Tronto suggests that the virtue, or "ethical quality," associated with the fifth phase of caring is solidarity. In order to "care with," we must demonstrate "solidarity," defined as "plurality, communication, trust and respect" (2013, p. 35), toward both those needing care and those providing it. Solidarity acknowledges the relational aspect of care and defines it as something in which we all might participate together. I believe that this means that the current inequities in care must be met by a commitment to providing care for those in need, and a recognition that caregivers must themselves be cared for—both of which are central principles of an ethic of care.

Perhaps the first changes can come from within the medical system, which can begin to assume more responsibility for the children it saves once they are home from the hospital. If we want to keep saving lives, which of course we do, we need to pay attention to the reality that care extends beyond merely meeting medical needs at home. This may be as inexpensive as rearranging medications to simplify the dosing schedule or enabling multiple specialty visits on the same day. It may be as simple as recognizing and supporting parental expertise. But some things will, of course, require more major changes in the system. Perhaps every family of a child with complex medical needs should be provided with a care coordinator who continues to aid in the arrangement of services at home. Perhaps pediatric centers need to establish regional, centralized home care, so that parents do not have to hire and train home health aides on their own. Perhaps some families need to be provided with supportive housing near to a pediatric center so that they can access services with less disruption to their lives.

As our population ages, and the process of moving health care into the home continues, we have been developing processes by which responsive care can be provided both for a dying person and for the family giving care. Hospice programs, for example, are expanding rapidly. These provide a wide range of support in the home, including appropriate medical equipment, medications, personal care, and, often, encouragement for family caregivers. Children with complex health care needs could be similarly supported in the home by a single agency that is prepared to take care of the multiplicity of the needs of both child and family. Perhaps programs to support extreme caregivers might grow out of the emerging pediatric and neonatal hospice movements. Given the complexity of the task, the enormous variability in children's medical problems, and the much longer time over which care is necessary, however, this will be a far more complicated process than providing hospice care.

Supporting the parents for whom extreme caregiving becomes a life-consuming process is essential. It is clear that care for many children is a round-the-clock necessity and that some, like Ian Brown's son Walker, cannot reasonably be cared for by only one or two people. While indeed parents are expected to give up some things in order to devote themselves to their children, it is not fair to ask them to permanently give up a career they desired and trained for, along with, for many, any prospect of financial security. It is also unfair to ask them to give up every moment of their personal time and all possibility of uninterrupted sleep. Many parent advocacy groups exist, but I know of none that are actively seeking legislation that would address this unfairness.

Financial support for caregivers is an absolute necessity. Parents like Brown are working a more-than-full-time job that is as taxing as any standard employment, yet they are not compensated for it or even considered to be working, though the work they are doing limits their ability to do paid work outside the home. Nonfamily home health care aides and other care workers receive minimal pay and even less respect, making caregiving undesirable as a career. We must promote caregiving as a respectable profession with training and adequate pay, whether it is being done by a family member or a hired home health care worker.

As Tronto suggests, political action will be required to bring about some changes. Indeed, positive change has already occurred in our educational system largely due to a political movement spearheaded by parents of disabled children. Their demand for equal education for children with disabilities paralleled the civil rights movement. The 1975 Individuals with Disabilities Education Act (IDEA) was a critical early step in civil rights legislation; it entitled all American children to a free public education appropriate to their specific needs. Following the Act, we as a nation have done fairly well creating opportunities within the educational system. It is not without problems but, despite ongoing battles over Individual Education Plans and lack of funding for programs, many extreme caregiving parents are supported by the extra developmental stimulation for their children and sometimes also benefit from the short break from their daily caregiving duties provided by the school day. Perhaps the Act was the first, tiny example of how a caring democracy might work.

But while school programs are enjoying at least partial success, once a child turns twenty-one, parents are once again on their own. Berube reports, "Most school districts simply keep kids with intellectual disabilities in high school until twenty-one, at which point the state has no more obligation to educate them" (2016, p. 150). And yet it is clear that developmental strides continue to be made in adulthood if there are responsive home and work environments. Forms of employment that provide the maximum amount of success in the least restrictive environment for an adult with intellectual disabilities are very hard to find. Employment programs geared toward people with intellecutal disabilities are often underfunded, and the work provided can be isolating and menial (Serres & Howatt, 2015). Children who have received an inclusive and affirming public education are dropped into a system that does not value them and often holds no place for them. Despite the years since the foundation of the first sheltered workshops in the 1970s, we still do not have satisfactory employment for many people with intellectual disabilities. Berube calls the creation of inclusive employment opportunities, "the next great civil rights struggle" (2016, p. 169). This could indeed be the focus of the next great legislation from our emerging caring democracy.

The possibility that a child might require extreme care, or even some care, for life should be recognized as well. We have seen that worries about the future loom large in the lives of extreme caregivers, particularly for the parents of children with intellectual disabilities. Parents cannot be required to continue caregiving into old age, nor should they be expected to be the only source of security and well-being when their children reach adulthood.

The establishment of homes away from home, allowing people with intellectual disabilities the freedom to move out, seems to me to be another urgent civil rights struggle. We need to end, or at least shorten, the wait list for placement, creating new homes so that parents know that there is an alternative available when needed. We may need to be creative about new forms of housing, perhaps including funding for larger houses or dormitory-style apartments. Of course, these homes will need to be staffed by caring individuals, so providing care workers with both higher pay and recognition for work done well is essential for success here as well.

I believe that continuing education, job creation, and guaranteed housing are the best places to invest our attention, advocacy, and political capital. We do not perhaps need to "live with" the intellectually disabled, as do the Brothers of Charity. Nor do we need to "work with" an intellectually disabled person at every workplace, though that might be nice. Tronto states, "It is possible to create responsive institutions that are staffed by people who are themselves attentive, responsible, competent, and responsive" (2013, p. 161). I believe the most important factor in long-term care for people with intellectual disabilities is to concentrate on educating the people who do care work to perform quiet listening and responsive caregiving so that the identity work started by parents can continue.

The promotion and encouragement of a caring democracy is in part a choice about what sort of society we wish to be. Our democracy, with its reliance on autonomy and personal choice may not be the easiest place to start, but Tronto believes it is possible to reshape America into a caring democracy. Perhaps thinking in terms of caring for each other might vastly improve our democracy and our society, by allowing us to imagine new ways of living (2013, p. 167). Perhaps we would all have less stress if we had the time to take care of ourselves and to pay attention to the needs of others. People who place a higher value on care than they do on, say, accumulating wealth, might be happier and healthier. We may indeed gain a better world if we integrated care into our public and private lives.

If we are to have a caring democracy, we as a society must learn to "care with" in solidarity with extreme caregiving parents. It seems to me that paying attention to the lessons of extreme caregivers would be a good place to start. We need to follow their example of becoming attentive to the multiple needs around us. We need to take responsibility for the care of both the special needs child and his or her parents. We need to practice listening to the sometimes quiet voices of those in need, and respond with care.

We might also personally benefit from learning the skills required to care for others, particularly the quiet listening necessary to become responsive to the needs of others. Those voices that are the hardest to hear might after all be the most important. John Green, author of the best-selling young adult novel *The Fault in Our Stars,* and video-blogging spokesperson for a generation of Millennials, recently gave a commencement speech at his alma mater, Kenyon College, which he titled "Learn to Listen." As he told an eager audience of college graduates,

> Living for one's self, even very successfully, will do absolutely nothing to fill the gasping void inside of you.
>
> In my experience, that void gets filled not through strength but through weakness. You must be weak before the world because love and listening weaken you. They make you vulnerable. They break you open. And it is only when you are weak that you can truly see and acknowledge and forgive and love the weakness in others. Weakness allows you to see other humans not as enemies to defeat, but as collaborators and co-creators. In the end, we're making humanness up together as we go along. (Green, 2016).

This is the lesson in humility and grace that parents learn by becoming extreme caregivers. During those sleepless nights, listening sometimes with desperate attention to determine their child's needs, they learn to understand and forgive weakness. They learn to live with dependency and vulnerability, in their child and in themselves. And they learn something about being human, making it up as they go along.

I hope this book has been the start of our journey to learn to listen to them.

REFERENCES

Albrecht, G. L. & Devlieger, P. J. (1999). The disability paradox: high quality of life against all odds. *Social Science and Medicine*, 48, 977–988.

Arras, John. (1997). Nice story but so what? Narrative and justification in ethics. In H. Lindemann Nelson (ed.), *Stories and their limits: narrative approaches to bioethics* (pp. 65–88). New York: Routledge.

Arras, J. D. & Dubler, N. N. (1994). Bringing the hospital home: ethical and social implications of high-tech home care. *The Hastings Center Report*, 24(5), S19–S28.

Baier, S. & Schomaker, M. Z. (1989). *Bed number ten*. Boca Raton, FL: CRC Press.

Bastek, T. K., Richardson, D. K., Zupancic, J. A. F., & Burns, J. P. (2005). Prenatal consultation practices at the border of viability: a regional survey. *Pediatrics*, 116, 407–413.

Beauchamp, T. L. & Childress, J. F. (2009). *Principles of biomedical ethics* (6th ed.). New York: Oxford University Press.

Berube, M. (1996). *Life as we know it: a father, a family, and an exceptional child*. New York: Pantheon Books, Random House.

Berube, M. (2016). *Life as Jamie knows it: an exceptional child grows up* (uncorrected proof). Boston, MA: Beacon Press.

Boss, R. D., Hutton, N., Sulpar, L. J., West, A. M., & Donohue, P.K. (2008). Values parents apply to decision-making regarding delivery room resuscitation for high-risk newborns. *Pediatrics*, 122, 583–589.

Bowden, P. (1998). Ethical attention: accumulating understandings. *European Journal of Philosophy*, 6(1), 59–77.

Boyd, R. (2004). Pity's pathologies portrayed: Rousseau and the limits of democratic compassion. *Political Theory*, 32, 519–546.

Braddock, D., Emerson, E., Felce, D., & Stancliffe, R. J. (2001). Living circumstances of children and adults with mental retardation or developmental disabilities in the United States, Canada, England and Wales, and Australia. *Mental Retardation and Developmental Disabilities Research Reviews*, 7, 115–121.

Bremer, A. (2007). The school of life. In K. L. Soper (ed.), *Gifts: mothers reflect on how children with Down syndrome enrich their lives* (pp. 87–90). Bethesda, MD: Woodbine House.

Brinchmann, B. S. (1999). When the home becomes a prison: living with a severely disabled child. *Nursing Ethics*, 6(2), 137–143.

Brody, H. (1997). Who gets to tell the story: narrative in postmodern bioethics. In H. Lindemann Nelson (ed.), *Stories and their limits: narrative approaches to bioethics* (pp. 18–30). New York: Routledge.

Brody, H. (2003). *Stories of sickness* (2nd ed.). New York: Oxford University Press.

Brody, H. & Clark, M. (2104). Narrative ethics: a narrative. *Narrative Ethics: The Role of Stories in Bioethics, special report, Hastings Center Report*, 44 (1), s7–s11.

Brown, I. (2011). *The boy in the moon: a father's journey to understand his extraordinary son*. New York: St Martin's Press.

Buck, P. S. (1950). *The child who never grew*. New York: John Day Company.

Callahan, S. (1988). The role of emotion in ethical decisionmaking. *Hastings Center Report*, 18(3), 9–24.

Caputo, J. D. (1993). *Against ethics: contributions to a poetics of obligation with constant reference to deconstruction*. Bloomington: Indiana University Press.

Carnevale, F. A., Alexander, E., Davis, M., Rennick, J., & Troini, R. (2006). Daily living with distress and enrichment: the moral experience of families with ventilator-assisted children at home. *Pediatrics*, 117(1), e48–e60.

Carver, L. (2007). My other half. In D. Brody (ed.), *The elephant in the playroom: ordinary parents write intimately and honestly about the extraordinary highs and heartbreaking lows of raising kids with special needs* (pp. 31–37). New York: Penguin.

Centers for Disease Control and Prevention (CDC). (2016). Prevalence and characteristics of autism spectrum disorder among children aged 8 years—autism and developmental disabilities monitoring network, 11 sites, United States, 2012. www.cdc.gov.

Chan, B., Jahnke, L,. Thorson, S., & Vanderburg, N. Minnesota Department of Health Division of Family Health (MDHDFH). (1998). *Caring for our children: a study of TEFRA in Minnesota, research by Minnesota children with special health needs*. http://www.mnddc.org/past/pdf/90s/98/98-DOH-TEFRA.pdf.

Christ, S. E. & Finger, S. (2004). Pearl S. Buck and Phenylketonuria. *The World of PKU*. www.pkuworld.org/home/historyprofile.

Cobb, A. D. (2016). Acknowledged dependence and the virtues of perinatal hospice. *Journal of Medicine and Philosophy*, 41(1), 25–40.

Cocchi, G., Gualdi, S., Bower, C., Halliday, J., Jonsson, B., Myrelid, A., & Doray, B. (2010). International trends of Down syndrome 1993–2004: births in relation to maternal age and terminations of pregnancies. *Birth Defects Research Part A: Clinical and Molecular Teratology*, 88(6), 474–479.

Cockett, A. (2012). Technology dependence and children: a review of the evidence. *Nursing Children and Young People*, 24(1), 32–35.

Corman, M. K. (2013). How mothers talk about placement of their child with autism outside the home. *Qualitative Health Research*, 23(10), 1320–1332.

Decker, J. (2011). *I wish I were engulfed in flames: my insane life raising two boys with autism* (Advance reader's copy). New York: Skyhorse.

Dybwik, K., Nielsen, E. W., & Brinchmann, B. S. (2011). Ethical challenges in home mechanical ventilation: a secondary analysis. *Nursing Ethics*, 19(2), 233–244.

Dyck, I., Konton, P., Angus, J., & McKeever, P. (2005). The home as a site for long-term care: meanings and management of bodies and spaces. *Health and Place*, 11, 173–185.

Edwards, S. D. (2009). Three versions of an ethics of care. *Nursing Philosophy*, 10, 231–240.

Egan, J. F., Benn, P. A., Zelop, C. M., Bolnick, A., Gianferrari, E., & Borgida, A. F. (2004). Down syndrome births in the United States from 1989 to 2001. *American Journal of Obstetrics and Gynecology*, 191(3), 1044–1048.

Elias, E. R. & Murphy, N. A. (2012). Home care of children and youth with complex health care needs and technology dependencies: a clinical report from the American Academy of Pediatrics (AAP). *Pediatrics*, 129(5), 996–1005.

Ehrenreich, B. (2010). *Bright-sided: how positive thinking is undermining America*. New York: Henry Holt.

Engber, D. (2015). The strange case of Anna Stubblefield. October 20, *New York Times Magazine*, www.nytimes.com.

Fadiman, A. (1997). *The spirit catches you and you fall down: a Hmong child, her American doctors, and the collision of two cultures*. New York: Farrar, Straus and Giroux.

Fei, D. (2015). *Girl in glass: how my "distressed baby" defied the odds, shamed a CEO, and taught me the essence of love, heartbreak, and miracles*. New York: Bloomsbury.

Feinberg, J. (1980). The child's right to an open future. In W. Aiken & H. LaFollette (eds.), *Whose child? Children's rights, parental authority, and state power* (pp. 124–153). Totowa, NJ: Rowman and Littlefield.

Field, D. J., Dorling, J. S., Manktelow, B. N., & Draper, E. S. (2008). Survival of extremely premature babies in a geographically defined population: prospective cohort study of 1994–9 compared with 2000–5. *BMJ*, 336(7655), 1221–1223.

Fins, J. J. (2006). *A palliative ethic of care: clinical wisdom at life's end*. Boston, MA: Jones and Bartlett.

Forman, V. (2009). *This lovely life: a memoir of premature motherhood*. New York: Houghton Mifflin Harcourt.

Fox, M. (2012). Lia Lee dies: life went on around her, redefining care. September 14, *New York Times*. www.nytimes.com.

Frank, A. (1995). *The wounded storyteller: body, illness, and ethics*. Chicago: University of Chicago Press.

Frank, A. (1997). Enacting illness stories: when, what, and why. In H. Lindemann Nelson (ed.), *Stories and their limits: narrative approaches to bioethics* (pp. 31–49). New York: Routledge.

Frank, A. W. (2002). "How can they act like that?" clinicians and patients as characters in each other's stories. *Hastings Center Report*, 32(6), 14–22.

Garden, R. (2010). Telling stories about illness and disability. *Perspectives in Biology and Medicine*, 52(1), 121–135.

Gilman, P. (2011). *The anti-romantic child: a story of unexpected joy*. New York: Harper Collins.

Goldberg, J. (2011). "Priority" waiting list to provide housing for thousands with developmental disabilities. April 17, *The Star-Ledger*. http://www.nj.com/news/index.ssf/2011/04/priority_waiting_list_to_provi.html.

Gray, R., Petrou, S., Hockley, C., & Gardner, F. (2007). Self-reported health status and health-related quality of life of teenagers who were born before 29 weeks' gestational age. *Pediatrics*, 120(1), e86–e93.

Grealy, L. (1994). *Autobiography of a face*. New York: Houghton Mifflin Company.

Green, J. (2016). Kenyon College: John Green commencement address. Kenyon College Video. https://www.youtube.com/watch?v=0AriZhzeHbA.

Green, S. E. (2003). "What do you mean 'what's wrong with her?' ": stigma and the lives of families of children with disabilities. *Social Science and Medicine*, 57, 1361–1374.

Green, S. E. (2006). "We're tired, not sad": benefits and burdens of mothering a child with a disability. *Social Science and Medicine*, 64, 150–163.

Greenfeld, J. (1970). *A child called Noah: a family journey*. New York: Harcourt Brace Jovanivich.

Greenfeld, J. (1978). *A place for Noah*. New York: Washington Square Press.

Greenfeld, J. (1986). *A client called Noah: a family journey continued*. New York: Henry Holt.

Greenfeld, K. T. (2009). *Boy alone: a brother's memoir*. New York: Harper Collins.

Greenfeld, K. T. (2009). Growing old with autism. May 25, *TIME*.

Groneberg, J. G. (2008). *Road map to Holland: how I found my way through my son's first two years with Down syndrome*. New York: New American Library.

Gunn, V. L. & Nechyba, C. (eds.). (2002). *The Harriet Lane handbook: a manual for pediatric house officers* (16th ed.). Philadelphia: Mosby Inc.

Hardwig, J. (1990). What about the family? *Hastings Center Report*, 20(2), 5–10.

Hardwig, J. (1997). Autobiography, biography, and narrative ethics. In H. Lindemann Nelson (ed.), *Stories and their limits: narrative approaches to bioethics* (pp. 50–64). New York: Routledge.

Harrison, H. (2001). Making lemonade: a parent's view of "quality of life" studies. *Journal of Clinical Ethics*, 12(3), 239–250.

Harrison, H. (2008). The offer they can't refuse: parents and perinatal treatment decisions. *Seminars in Fetal and Neonatal Medicine*, 13, 329–334.

Hart, C. (1989). *Without reason: a family copes with two generations of autism*. New York: Harper and Rowe.

Huffman, J. S. (2007). It's better than good. In K. L. Soper (ed.), *Gifts: mothers reflect on how children with Down syndrome enrich their lives* (pp. 38–43). Bethesda, MD: Woodbine House.

Iversen, P. (2006). *Strange son: two mothers, two sons, and the quest to unlock the hidden world of autism*. New York: Riverhead Books.

Jennings, A. (1995). My heart child: a portrait of Savannah: life lessons learned from an infant with chronic illness. Unpublished.

Keenan, H. T., Doron, M. W., & Seyda, B. A. (2005). Comparison of mothers' and counselors' perceptions of predelivery counseling for extremely premature infants. *Pediatrics*, 116, 104–111.

Kirk, S. (1998). Families' experiences of caring at home for a technology-dependent child: a review of the literature. *Child: Care, Health and Development*, 24(2), 101–114.

Kirk, S., Glendinning, C., & Callery, P. (2005). Parent or nurse? the experience of being the parent of a technology-dependent child. *Journal of Advanced Nursing*, 51(5), 456–464.

Kittay, E. (1999). *Love's labor: essays on women, equality, and dependency.* New York: Routledge.

Kittay, E. (2010). Planning a trip to Italy, arriving in Holland: the delusion of choice in planning a family. *IJFAB: International Journal of Feminist Approaches to Bioethics*, 3(2), 9–24.

Kittay, E. (2011). Forever small: the strange case of Ashley X. *Hypatia*, 26(3), 610–631.

Kosho, T., Nakamura, T., Kawame, H., Baba, A., Tamura, M., & Fukushima, Y. (2006). Neonatal management of trisomy 18: clinical details of 24 patients receiving intensive treatment. *American Journal of Medical Genetics Part A*, 140A, 937–944.

Kuo, D. Z., Cohen, E., Agrawal, R. Berry, J. G., & Casey, P. H. (2011). A national profile of caregiver challenges among more medically complex children with special health care needs. *Archives of Pediatric and Adolescent Medicine*, 165 (11), 1020–1026.

Lalvani, P. (2011). Constructing the (m)other: dominant and contested narratives on mothering a child with Down syndrome. *Narrative Inquiry*, 21(2), 276–293.

Landsman, G. H. (1998). Reconstructing motherhood in the age of "perfect" babies: mothers of infants and toddlers with disabilities. *Journal of Women in Culture and Society*, 24(1), 69–99.

Landsman, G. H. (1999). Does God give special kids to special parents? personhood and the child with disabilities as gift and as giver. In L. L. Layne (ed.), *Transformative motherhood: on giving and getting in a consumer culture* (pp. 133–165). New York: New York University Press.

Lantos, J. D. & Kohrman, A. F. (1992). Ethical aspects of pediatric home care. *Pediatrics*, 80(5), 920–924.

Layne, L. L. (1999). The child as gift: new directions in the study of Euro-American gift exchange. In L. L. Layne (ed.), *Transformative motherhood: on giving and getting in a consumer culture* (pp. 1–27). New York: New York University Press.

Leone, M. (2010). *Knowing Jesse: a mother's story of grief, grace, and everyday bliss.* New York: Simon and Schuster.

Lindahl, B., Sandman, P. O., & Rasmussen, B. H. (2006). On being dependent on home mechanical ventilation: depictions of patients' experiences over time. *Qualitative Health Research*, 17(7), 881–901.

Lindemann, H. (2009). Holding one another (well, wrongly, clumsily) in a time of dementia. *Metaphilosophy*, 40(3–4), 416–424.

Lindemann Nelson, H. (1997). Introduction. In H. Lindemann Nelson (ed.), *Stories and their limits: narrative approaches to bioethics* (pp. vii–xx). New York: Routledge.

Lindemann Nelson, H. (2004). Four narrative approaches to bioethics. In G. Khushf (ed.), *Handbook of bioethics: taking stock of the field from a philosophical perspective* (pp. 163–181). Springer Netherlands.

Lindemann Nelson, H. (2014). *Holding and letting go: the social practice of personal identities.* New York: Oxford University Press.

Macnaughton, J. (2009). The dangerous practice of empathy. *The Lancet*, 373 (June 6), 1940–1941.

Malek, J. (2009). What really is in a child's best interest? Toward a more precise picture of the interests of children. *Journal of Clinical Ethics*, 20(2), 175–182.

Mansell, J. (2006). Deinstitutionalisation and community living: progress, problems and priorities. *Journal of Intellectual and Developmental Disability*, 31(2), 65–76.

Marlow, N., Wolke, D., Bracewell, M.A., & Samara, M. (2005). Neurologic and developmental disability at six years of age after extremely preterm birth. *New England Journal of Medicine*, 352(1), 9–19.

Mattingly, C. (2014). *Moral laboratories: family peril and the struggle for a good life.* Oakland: University of California Press.

McArthur, P. (2012). Carried and held: getting good at being helped. *International Journal of Feminist Approaches to Bioethics*, 5(2), 162–169.

McGraw, M. P. & Perlman, J. M. (2008). Attitudes of neonatologists toward delivery room management of confirmed Trisomy 18: potential factors influencing a changing dynamic. *Pediatrics*, 121(6), 1106–1110.

McKeever, P. & Miller, K.-L. (2004). Mothering children who have disabilities: a Bourdieusian interpretation of maternal practices. *Social Science and Medicine*, 59, 1177–1191.

Mercurio, M. R. (2005). Physicians' refusal to resuscitate at borderline gestational age. *Journal of Perinatology*, 25, 685–689.

Montross, C. (2007). *Body of work: meditations on mortality from the human anatomy lab.* New York: Penguin Press.

Morrice, P. (2009). The normal one. June 3, *New York Times*. www.nytimes.com.

Morris, J. K. & Alberman, E. (2009). Trends in Down's syndrome live births and antenatal diagnoses in England and Wales from 1989 to 2008: analysis of data from the National Down Syndrome Cytogenetic Register. *BMJ*, 339, b3794.

Natoli, J. L., Ackerman, D. L., McDermott, S., & Edwards, J. G. (2012). Prenatal diagnosis of Down syndrome: a systematic review of termination rates (1995–2011). *Prenatal diagnosis*, 32(2), 142–153.

Neuwirth, Z. E. (1997). Physician empathy—should we care? *The Lancet*, 350 (Aug. 30), 606.

Noddings, N. (1984). *Caring: a feminine approach to ethics and moral education.* Berkeley: University of California Press.

Noddings, N. (1994). Moral obligation or moral support for high-tech home care? *Hastings Center Report,* 24(5, special supplement), S6–S10.

O'Higgins, B. (2011). Wait is long for disability services. September 1, KMUW Radio, transcribed at End the Wait Kansas. http://www.endthewaitks.org/news/wait-is-long-for-disability-services.

Pistorius, M. (2013). *Ghost boy: the miraculous escape of a misdiagnosed boy trapped inside his own body.* Nashville, TN: Harper Collins Christian.

Price, B. (2007). When the other shoe drops. In K. L. Soper (ed.), *Gifts: mothers reflect on how children with down syndrome enrich their lives* (pp. 187–192). Bethesda, MD: Woodbine House.

Rapp, E. (2013). *The still point of the turning world.* New York: Penguin Press.

Rapp, E. (2013). NPR audio interview. March 18. http://www.NPR.org/books/titles/174114011/the-still-point-of-the-turning-world.

Ray, L. D. (2002). Parenting and childhood chronicity: making visible the invisible work. *Journal of Pediatric Nursing*, 17(6), 424–438.

Rizzo, M. (2014). Why we published a photo of a 16-year-old in a diaper. July 10, *Shots: Health News from NPR.* www.NPR.org.

Romley, J. A., Shah, A. K., Chung, P. J., Elliott, M. N., Vestal, K. D., & Schuster, M. A. (2017). Family-provided health care for children with special health care needs. *Pediatrics*, 139(1), e20161287.

Saigal, S., Feeny, D., Rosenbaum, P., Furlong, W., Burrows, E., & Stoskopf, B. (1996). Self-perceived health status and health-related quality of life of extremely low-birth-weight infants at adolescence. *Journal of the American Medical Association*, 276(6), 453–459.

Saigal, S., Stoskopf, B. I., Feeny, D., Furlong, W., Burrows, E., Rosenbaum, P. I., & Hoult, L. (1999). Differences in preferences for neonatal outcomes among health professionals, parents, and adolescents. *Journal of the American Medical Association*, 281(21), 1991–1997.

Saigal, S., Stoskopf, B. I., Streiner, D. I., & Burrows, E. (2001). Physical growth and current health status of infants who were of extremely low birth weight and controls at adolescence. *Pediatrics*, 108(2), 407–415.

Sea, S. (2003). Planet autism. September 27. *salon.com*. http://www.salon.com/2003/09/27/autism.

Seltzer, M. M. & Krauss, W. M. (2001). Quality of life of adults with mental retardation/developmental disabilities who live with family. *Mental Retardation and Developmental Disabilities Research Reviews*, 7(2), 105–114.

Serres, C. & Howatt, G. (2015). Dead-end jobs, low pay. November 8, *Minneapolis Star Tribune*. www.startribune.com.

Sharot, T. (2011). *The optimism bias: a tour of the irrationally positive brain*. New York: Pantheon Books.

Shaw, K., Cartwright, C., & Craig, J. (2011). The housing and support needs of people with an intellectual disability into older age. *Journal of Intellectual Disability Research*, 55(9), 895–903.

Simon, R. (2002). *Riding the bus with my sister: a true life journey*. New York: Houghton Mifflin.

Slomka, J. (1992). The negotiation of death: clinical decision making at the end of life. *Social Science and Medicine*, 35(3), 251–259.

Slote, M. (2007). *The ethics of care and empathy*. New York: Routledge.

Smith, T. (1999). *Miracle birth stories of very premature babies: little thumbs up!* Westport, CT: Bergin and Garvey.

Solomon, A. (2012). *Far from the tree: parents, children, and the search for identity*. New York: Scribner.

Soper, K. L. (ed.). (2007). *Gifts: mothers reflect on how children with Down syndrome enrich their lives*. Bethesda, MD: Woodbine House.

Spink, K. (1991). *Jean Vanier & L'Arche: a communion of love*. New York: Crossroad.

Stainton, T., Brown, J., Crawford, C., Hole, R., & Charles, G. (2011). Comparison of community residential supports on measures of information & planning; access to & delivery of supports; choice & control; community connections; satisfaction; and, overall perception of outcomes. *Journal of Intellectual Disability Research*, 55(8), 732–745.

Steinmetz, K. (2015). Help! My parents are Millennials. October 26, *TIME*.

Streiner, D. L., Saigal, S., Burrows, E., Stoskopf, B., & Rosenbaum, P. (2001). Attitudes of parents and health care professionals toward active treatment of extremely premature infants. *Pediatrics*, 108(1), 152–157.

Tarabay, J. (2010). Haunted house has painful past as an asylum. October 29, *NPR News*. www.NPR.org.

Terruwe, A. A. A. & Kroft, A. L. (2006). *Crossing the barrier: modern visions on care for humanising mentally disabled people*. Gent, Belgium: Brothers of Charity.

Thomson, J., Shah, S. S., Simmons, J. M., Sauers-Ford, H. S., Brunswick, S., Hall, D., Kahn, R. S., & Beck, A. F. (2016). Financial and social hardships in families of children with medical complexity. *Journal of Pediatrics*, 172, 187–193.

Tronto, J. (1993). *Moral boundaries: a political argument for an ethic of care.* New York: Routledge.

Tronto, J. (2013). *Caring democracy: markets, equality, and justice.* New York: New York University Press.

Trute, B., Benzies, K. M., Worthington, C., Reddon, J. R., & Moore, M. (2010). Accentuate the positive to mitigate the negative: mother psychological coping resources and family adjustment in childhood disability. *Journal of Intellectual and Developmental Disability*, 35(1), 36–43.

Ubel, P. A., Schwarz, N., Loewenstein, G., & Smith, D. (2005). Misimagining the unimaginable: the disability paradox and health care decision making. *Health Psychology*, 24(4), S57–S62.

Volbrecht, R. M. (2002). *Nursing ethics: communities in dialogue.* Upper Saddle River, NJ: Prentice Hall:.

Walker, M. U. (1992). Feminism, ethics, and the question of theory. *Hypatia*, 7(3), 23–38.

Wang, K. W. K. & Bernard, A. (2004). Technology-dependent children and their families: a review. *Journal of Advanced Nursing*, 45(1), 36–46.

Weeks, L. E., Nilsson, T., Bryanton, O., & Kozma, A. (2009). Current and future concerns of older parents with sons and daughters with intellectual disabilities. *Journal of Policy and Practice in Intellectual Disabilities*, 6(3), 180–188.

Weiss, A. R., Binns, H. J., Collins Jr., J. W., & deRegnier, R.-A. (2007). Decision-making in the delivery room: a survey of neonatologists. *Journal of Perinatology*, 27, 754–760.

Wilkinson, D. J. (2011). Shedding light on the gray zone. *American Journal of Bioethics*, 11(2), W3–W5.

Woodwell, W. H. (2001). *Coming to term: a father's story of birth, loss, and survival.* Mississippi: University Press of Mississippi.

Wright, P. (2010). The history of special education law. November 29. www.wrightslaw.com.

Wynn, F. (2002). Nursing and the concept of life: towards and ethics of testimony. *Nursing Philosophy*, 3, 120–132.

Zibricky, C. D. (2014). New knowledge about motherhood: an autoethnography on raising a disabled child. *Journal of Family Studies*, 20(1), 39–47.

INDEX

AAP. *See* American Academy of Pediatrics
Abortion, 28, 29, 96, 104, 105
Action, caring as, 76, 78, 81, 87, 93, 124
Advocacy, 9, 53, 63, 96, 110–16, 222.
   See also Value, maintenance of
"Against Ethics" (Caputo), 81
Albrecht, G. L., 61
Alzheimer's disease, in Down syndrome, 196–97
Ambivalence, 96, 103–10
American Academy of Pediatrics (AAP), guidelines for discharge, 85, 86, 130, 132
Americans with Disabilities Act, 216
Annette (mother of individual with CFC), ix–xvii, 3, 40, 174–75. *See also* Savannah
Anti-Romantic Child, The (Gilman), 141. *See also* Gilman, Benjamin; Gilman, Priscilla
Apnea monitors, 71, 80
Applied behavioral analysis, 145. *See also* Operant conditioning
Aristotle, 73, 76
Arras, John, 65, 119
Association for Retarded Children, 203
Attentiveness, 75, 76–77, 78–81, 94–123, 124, 222. *See also* Advocacy; Ambivalence; Choice, perceived lack of; Uncertainty
  extremes of, 79–80
  ideal of, 79
  long-term care arrangements and, 213
  responsibility and, 83, 94–95
Autism, xviii, 23, 31, 58, 59, 106, 197. *See also* Greenfeld, Noah; Hart, Sumner; Hart, Ted; Iversen, Dov; Jack; Tito
  avoidance of term, 141
  financial burden of care and, 44–45
  guilt experienced by parents, 99, 211–12
  incidence of, 26
  long-term care arrangements and, 198, 211–12
  physical burden of care and, 39, 43
  quest for knowledge on, 137, 138–39, 141, 145–47, 148–49, 152–53
  responsiveness and, 163–68, 172, 178, 182–83
  social isolation and, 50–51, 52, 53, 54–55
Autobiography of a Face (Grealy), 34
Autonomy, 72, 116–17. *See also* Independence

Baby Doe laws, 67, 69
Baier, Sue, 158
Beauchamp, Tom, 67, 72
Bed Number Ten (Baier and Schomaker), 158
Beneficence, 67, 68

241

Berube, Jamie, 114, 171, 196–97, 200, 205–6, 210. *See also* Berube, Michael
Berube, Michael, 225
  on education, 229
  on long-term care arrangements, 196–97, 200, 201, 202, 205–6
  quest for knowledge, 143–44, 147
  on value of son, 114, 210
Best interests of the child standard, 4–5, 7, 67–68, 69, 72, 118–19, 121, 188
Bioethics. *See* Ethics
Blindness, 20, 22, 70, 128, 143
Body of Work (Montross), 181
Bowden, Peta, 79
Boy Alone (Greenfeld, K. T.), 34n2, 45, 106
Boy in the Moon, The: A Father's Journey to Understand His Extraordinary Son (Brown), 8–9, 36–37, 55, 100, 102, 135, 136, 172, 175–76, 201. *See also* Brown, Ian; Brown, Walker
Boy Scouts of America (special-needs troops), 203, 207. *See also* Eagle Scouts
Bremer, A., 116, 136, 139
Brinchmann, Berit, 52, 104, 105, 120
Brody, Howard, 58, 64, 65, 160–61
Brothers of Charity, 203, 215, 216, 217, 220, 230
Brown, Ian, 8–9, 155, 181, 209, 224, 228
  ambivalence of, 107–8, 109
  feelings of failure, 148–52, 156
  guilt experienced by, 99–100
  on lack of choice, 120
  on long-term care arrangements, 197, 200, 201, 202, 211, 212–13
  on negativity silencing, 59, 62–63
  on physical burden of care, 36–37, 38
  quest for knowledge, 135, 136, 139–41, 142, 144–45, 146
  responsibility and, 99–100, 101, 102–3
  responsiveness and, 171, 172–73, 175–76, 178–79, 182, 183–84, 185, 190
  self-disparagement of, 146
  on social isolation, 55
Brown, Johanna, 171, 183–84

Brown, Walker, 36–37, 39, 55, 62–63, 99–100, 101, 102–3, 107–8, 135, 139–41, 142, 146, 149–52, 153, 155, 168, 171, 172–73, 174, 175–76, 178–79, 182, 183, 185, 186, 190, 197, 200, 201, 209, 211, 212–13, 217, 224, 228. *See also* Brown, Ian
Buck, Carol, 211
Buck, Pearl S., 211

CAN. *See* Cure Autism Now
Cancer, in children, 22, 151
Caputo, John, 81
Cardiofaciocutaneous syndrome (CFC), 39, 59, 102. *See also* Brown, Walker; Greenhaw, Kinley; Lydicksen, Luke; Savannah
  quest for knowledge on, 139–41, 142, 144–45, 146, 152
  rarity of, 36, 139
  responsiveness and, 171, 172–73, 174–75, 177–78, 181, 182
Care ethics/ethic of care, 10, 11, 12, 14, 73, 74, 79, 81, 93, 148, 223, 227. *See also* Noddings, Nel; Phases of Care; Tronto, Joan
Caregiving
  care for providers of, 9–10, 12, 227, 228
  funding for encouraged, 225
  knowledge and expertise of providers, 127, 144–45, 153
  narrative of, 70–72
  promoting as a profession, 228
  self-disparagement of providers, 145–48
  training of providers, 125–26
  value of unrecognized, 9, 49–50
Care-giving (phase of care), 94, 124
  defined, 75
  process of, 83–86
  virtue associated with (*see* Competence)
Care-receiving (phase of care), 94, 157
  defined, 75
  process of, 86–93

virtue associated with (*see*
  Responsiveness)
Caring about (phase of care), 94, 124
  defined, 75
  process of, 78–81
  virtue associated with (*see*
    Attentiveness)
"Caring bridge" sites, 33
Caring Democracy (Tronto), 77,
  185–86, 226–27
Caring with (phase of care), 77, 226–31
Carnevale, F. A., 32, 39, 43, 48, 53, 54,
  98, 105
CDLS. *See* Cornelia DeLang syndrome
Center for Disease Control and Prevention
  (CDC), 26
Cerebral palsy, 20, 22, 42–43, 60, 71, 98
CFC. *See* Cardiofaciocutaneous syndrome
Chaos narratives, 58
Child Called Noah, A: A Family Journey
  (Greenfeld), 44–45, 106, 135,
  136. *See also* Greenfeld, Josh;
  Greenfeld, Noah
Child protection laws, 124–25
Child Protection Services, 133
Children with special health care needs
  (CSHCN), 26, 45, 47, 48, 118
Childress, James, 67, 72
Choice, perceived lack of, 96, 116–21
Client Called Noah, A (Greenfeld), 45
Cobb, Aaron, 226
Colic, 173–74
Communication problems, 22–23. *See
  also* Nonverbal children; Tito
Community. *See also* Support systems
  and programs
  encouraging involvement of, 202,
    206–10, 226–31
  expressive-collaborative model on, 73
Competence, 75, 76–77, 83–86, 94,
  124–56, 223
  lack of, 124–25, 132
  lack of recognized standards for, 85
  measuring, 125, 126–34
  medical definition of, 130
  professional, 83–84

quest for knowledge and, 134–56
responsiveness and, 158
Complex medical needs, 21–22. *See also*
  Children with special health care
  needs; Medical complexity; Medical
  fragility
Cornelia DeLang syndrome (CDLS),
  xvii–xviii, 4, 23, 40, 226
  average age of fatality, xvii
  child's identity and, 170
  social isolation and, 52
Cost of care, 118, 209, 216. *See also*
  Financial burden of care
CSHCN. *See* Children with special health
  care needs
Cure Autism Now (CAN), 145, 164

Dangerous behavior, 40–41, 43, 199–200
Deafness/hearing loss, 20, 22, 23, 128
Death. *See also* Withholding treatment
  ambivalence toward, 103–10
  letting go and, 186–91
  murder/suicide fantasy, 105–8
Decision Enterprises Corporation
  (DEC), 203–4
Dementia, in Down syndrome, 160, 161
Dependency
  changing thinking on, 227
  ethics and, 73
  extreme, 10, 159
  total, 20
  utter, 11
Devlieger, P. J., 61
Diagnosis
  coming to terms with, 137–38
  as identity, 169–73
  research into, 137–42
Diaper changes, 40, 42–43
Didion, Joan, 144
Disability
  defining, 18–23
  mild, 20, 21, 28
  moderate, 20–21, 28
  multiple severe, 25–26, 27
  severe, 20, 28
Disability paradox, 61–62

Down syndrome, x, 19, 23, 31, 58, 207, 218, 225. *See also* Berube, Jamie; Groneberg, Avery; Price, Jude
    blaming of parents for, 112
    the child's identity and, 171
    long-term care arrangements and, 195–97, 200, 205–6, 214
    perceived lack of care choices, 120
    quest for knowledge on, 135–36, 137–38, 143–44, 147
    rate of, 29
    screening for, 29, 112
    valuing children with, 114, 115–16

Eagle Scouts, 195, 207–10
Education, 56–57, 229, 230
    laws establishing right to, 56n3
    parental responsibility for, 95–96
    social isolation in, 52
Education for All Handicapped Children Act of 1975, 56n3
Edwards, Steve, 78
Elementary and Secondary Education Act of 1965, 56n3
Emotions, 13–14, 73, 76
    attentiveness and, 78–79
    competence and, 83, 84–85
    mirroring of, 90
    responsiveness and, 87, 88, 89, 91
Employment
    relinquishing of, 35, 47, 49–50
    for special-needs individuals, 202, 203–6, 229, 230
End the Wait Kansas, 198
Epilepsy, 22, 71. *See also* Seizures
Ethics, 4–5, 14, 64–93, 116
    care (*see* Care ethics/ethic of care)
    expressive-collaborative model, 73
    feminist, 11, 73
    of genetic testing, 30
    literature on, 32
    narrative, 58, 64–72
    phases of care (*see* Phases of care)
    principles of, 67–68, 72
    theoretical-juridical model, 73
    virtue, 73, 76, 223

Expressive-collaborative model, 73
Extreme caregiving
    categories of need requiring, 21–23
    defining, 11–14
    number of families involved in, 30
    overlooked in medical records, 2
    parenting *vs.*, 14–18
    quantifying, 23–27
    statistics, 27–31
Extreme dependency, 10, 159

Facilitated communication, 165, 179
Fadiman, Ann, 41–42, 132. *See also* Lee, Fuoa; Lee, Lia
Failure, facing, 148–56
Far From the Tree (Solomon), 25
Fathers, and gendered nature of caregiving, 34–35
Feedback loop, caregiving as, 84, 86–87, 91, 93, 157, 189
Fei, Deanna, 46–47, 143, 188
Feinberg, Joel, 17, 162
Feminism, 49, 79
Feminist ethics, 11, 73
Financial burden of care, 44–50. *See also* Cost of care
Fins, Joseph J., 15
Forman, Ellie, 67, 68–69, 71, 72, 82, 83
Forman, Evan, 67, 70–73, 82–83, 85, 92–93. *See also* Forman, Vicky
Forman, Vicky, 66–73, 74
    attentiveness and, 80
    competence and, 85–86
    narrative of caregiving, 70–72
    narrative of premature birth, 66–70
    quest for knowledge, 143, 146
    responsibility and, 82–83
    responsiveness and, 92–93
    self-disparagement of, 146
Frank, Arthur, 65, 89, 158, 160–61, 180–81
Freitag, Paul, xiv–xvii, 3, 6, 27, 34, 168, 192–95, 196, 198–99, 202–10
    birth of, xiv
    developmental level of, 19–20, 21, 194
    diagnosis of, 19, 193

as an Eagle Scout, 195, 207–10
education of, 52, 56–57
employment of, 203–6
family involvement in care, xv
father's death, 217–19
father's relationship with, 56–57, 59, 62, 63, 101–2, 103, 105–6, 109, 154, 203
friend's death, 218
institutionalization suggested for, xiv, 9, 117
living arrangements of, 213, 214–21
mother's devotion to, xiv–xv, xvii, 54, 218–19
probable cause of disabilities, xv
social isolation of, 52–53
in Special Olympics, 195, 203, 206–7
withholding of treatment suggested for, 101–2, 103
Future. *See* Long-term care arrangements

Gastrostomy-tube feeding, xi, xiii, xiv–xv, 16, 36, 37, 39, 128, 130
Genetic testing, 29–30, 112, 137, 152. *See also* Prenatal screening
Ghost Boy (Pistorius), 34, 158–59
Gifts: Mothers Reflect on How Children with Down Syndrome Enrich Their Lives (Soper, ed.), 114, 137, 196
Gifts narrative, 113–15
Gilman, Benjamin, 141
Gilman, Priscilla, 141, 182–83
Girl in Glass (Fei), 46–47. *See also* Fei, Dianna
Grealy, Lucy, 34
Green, John, 231
Green, Sara, 33, 60, 98, 100, 115
Greenfeld, Josh
  ambivalence of, 106–7, 109
  feelings of failure, 149–50, 156
  on financial burden of care, 44–45
  guilt experienced by, 99
  on lack of choice, 120–21
  on long-term care arrangements, 199–200
  on negativity silencing, 63
  quest for knowledge, 135, 136, 138–39, 140, 145
  responsibility and, 99, 100–101
  responsiveness and, 172, 177
  self-disparagement of, 145
  on social isolation, 54–55
Greenfeld, Karl Taro, 34n2, 45, 54, 106
Greenfeld, Noah, 44–45, 50, 54–55, 63, 99, 100–101, 106–7, 120–21, 138–39, 140, 145, 149–50, 168, 177, 199–200, 210. *See also* Greenfeld, Josh
Greenhaw, Kinley (child with CFC), 182
Greenhaw, Shelly, 182
Grey zone, in prematurity, 67, 69
Grief, 98, 137, 144, 211, 212, 213
Groneberg, Avery (child with Down syndrome), 171
Groneberg, Jennifer Graf, x, 171
G-tube feeding. *See* Gastrostomy-tube feeding
Guillain-Barré syndrome, 158
Guilt, 96, 97, 99–100, 103, 138, 211–12, 213

HALO: Helping Autism through Learning and Outreach, 168n1
Hardwig, John, 5
Harm standard, 16, 68, 69, 124–25
  incompetence, 131–34
Harriet Lane Handbook, 28
Harrison, Helen, 59–60, 61, 69, 110
Hart, Charles
  ambivalence of, 106, 107, 109
  feelings of failure, 152–53, 156
  guilt experienced by, 99
  on long-term care arrangements, 211, 212
  murder/suicide fantasy of, 106
  on positive thinking, 59
  quest for knowledge, 135, 140, 141, 146–47
  responsiveness and, 172, 178, 182
  on social isolation, 50–51, 52
Hart, Sumner, 52, 56, 106, 107, 210, 211
Hart, Ted, 50–51, 106, 140, 141, 146–47, 152–53, 178, 186, 211, 212. *See also* Hart, Charles

Health and Human Services Department, 198
Hearing loss. *See* Deafness/hearing loss
Heart problems, xvii, 4, 128, 135
Hmong culture, 41–42, 133
Holding in an identity, 160, 169, 189, 201, 223
Hospice, 226, 228
Hospitalization, 117–18, 119–20
Hyperlexia with sensory integration dysfunction, 141
Hypersensitivity to stimuli, 141
Hypoxic-ischemic encephalopathy, xv

IDEA (Individuals with Disabilities Education Act), 229
Identity, 17, 159–63. *See also* Life story
 disability/disease impact on, 169–73
 formation of, 160–63
 holding in an, 160, 169, 189, 201, 223
IEPs. *See* Individual Education Plans
Independence, 16–17, 20–21, 155. *See also* Autonomy
Individual Education Plans (IEPs), 95, 229
Individual Service Plans (ISPs), 21, 216, 220–21
Individuals with Disabilities Education Act (IDEA), 229
Infantile spasms, 71, 92–93, 146
Innovative Technology for Autism (CAN conference), 164
Institutions/institutionalization, 120–21. *See also* Out-of-home placement
 abuses in, xiv, 107, 199, 210–11
 parents urged to consider, xiv, 9, 117
 successful placement, 211
Insurance. *See* Medical insurance
Intellectual disability, 22, 60, 85
Interdependence, 73, 77
IQ scores, 19, 20, 21
ISPs. *See* Individual Service Plans
Iversen, Dov, 163–64, 167–68. *See also* Iversen, Portia
Iversen, Portia
 quest for knowledge, 145–46
 responsiveness and, 163–64, 166, 167–68, 172

Jack (individual with autism), 148–49, 153, 197–98
Jeanette (child with special needs), 96–97, 103, 186–87
John, Brother (Brothers of Charity), 215–16, 217, 218, 220
Journal of the American Medical Association, 59
Justice, 67

Kingsley, Emily Perl, ix. *See also* "Welcome to Holland"
Kirk, Susan, 13, 16, 24, 32, 38, 45, 47, 48, 51, 98, 118, 128, 131
Kittay, Eva Feder, 10, 11–12, 176–77, 182, 183
Kittay, Sesha (individual with special needs), 11, 12, 176–77
Knowledge, quest for, 134–56. *See also* Quest narratives
Kometani, Foumi, 44–45, 177

Landsman, Gail, 33, 112–13, 114, 120
Lantos, John, 119
L'Arche, 201–2, 203, 206, 213, 217, 220
Lee, Foua, 41–42
Lee, Lia, 41–42, 43, 63, 132–33
Leukemia, 136
Levin, Dana, 144
Life as Jamie Knows It (Berube), 205–6
Life As We Know It: A Father, a Family, and an Exceptional Child (Berube), 143–44, 205. *See also* Berube, Jamie; Berube, Michael
Life story, 17, 158, 189–90, 223. *See also* Identity
 creation of, 160–63
 disability/disease impact on, 170
 for nonverbal children, 173–80
Linda (mother of child with CDLS), xvii–xviii, 3, 49–50. *See also* Samuel
Lindahl, Berit, 84
Lindemann, Hilde, 17, 65, 160, 161, 188–89
Listening, quiet, 220–21
Long-term care arrangements, 6, 192–221
 community involvement in, 202, 206–10, 229–30

employment, 202, 203–6, 229, 230
out-of-home placement (*see* Out-of-home placement)
preparations, 195–203
Lovass, Ivar, 145
Love, 70, 92, 179, 185
Love's Labor (Kittay), 11–12
Lydicksen, Angie, 177, 179, 180
Lydicksen, Luke (child with CFC), 177

McKeever, P., 47, 54, 174
Macnaughton, Jane, 90
Maleficence, 68
Malek, J., 5, 14, 125
MARC. *See* Montgomery County Association for Retarded Children
Marlow, Neil, 20–21, 28
Mattingly, Cheryl, 91, 108–9, 118, 121, 127, 132
MDHDFH. *See* Minnesota Department of Health, Division of Family Health
Medical complexity, 45
Medical fragility, 15
Medical insurance, 45, 46–47
Medical system. *See also* Physicians
caregiving responsibilities unrecognized by, 9
challenges caused by advances in, 4, 30
changes suggested for, 227–28
disillusionment with, 150–53
expectations of cures and treatment, 30, 224–25
language of, 139–43
parents' relationships with, 142–43
refusing advice of, 85
responsibility of, 82–83, 126
"Mental retardation," 19–20, 193
Mental retardation or developmental disabilities (MR/DD), 196, 198
Mild disability, 20, 21, 28
Miller, K.-L., 54, 174
Minnesota Department of Health, Division of Family Health (MDHDFH), 24–25
Moderate disability, 20–21, 28
Montgomery County Association for Retarded Children (MARC), 56–57, 198–99

Montgomery County Department of Developmental Disabilities and Behavioral Health (MCDDDBH), 216
Montross, Christine, 181
Moral Boundaries: A Political Argument for an Ethic of Care (Tronto), 73. *See also* Phases of care; Tronto, Joan
Mothers
ambivalence in, 108–9
employment relinquished by, 35, 47, 50
guilt experienced by, 211–12
knowledge and expertise of, 127, 144–45
level of care provided by, 34–35
"perfect baby," expectations for, 111–13
MR/DD. *See* Mental retardation or developmental disabilities
Mukhopadhyay, Tito, 168n1. *See also* Tito
Multiple severe disability (MSD), 25–26, 27
Murder/suicide fantasy, 105–8

Narratives, 33–63
of caregiving, 70–72
chaos, 58
of child's life (*see* Life story)
ethical analysis, 58, 64–72
on financial burden of care, 44–50
of gifts, 113–15
on negativity silencing, 56–63
on physical burden of care, 36–43
of premature birth, 66–70
quest (*see* Quest narratives)
redemptive, 58
on social isolation, 50–56
of specialness, 113, 115
National Public Radio, 104
Negativity silencing, 56–63
Neonatal intensive care unit (NICU) survivors, 18, 20, 59–60, 120
Neonatology, advances in, 27–29
New Jersey Star-Ledger, 198
NICU. *See* Neonatal intensive care unit
Noddings, Nel, 34, 38, 87, 89, 91
Nonmaleficience, 67

Nonverbal children, 172, 173–80, 223.
　　See also Communication problems

Open future, right to, 17, 162
Operant conditioning, 44, 107, 145
Out-of-home placement, 198–202,
　　210–21. See also Institutions/
　　institutionalization
　　advantages of, 213–14
　　guilt caused by, 211–12, 213
　　improvements suggested for, 230
　　statistics for, 198
　　successful outcome determinants, 219
　　wait lists, 198, 213, 230

"Parenting plus," 15, 39, 42–43
Paternalism, 78, 84
Patterning, 44
Paul (author's brother). See Freitag, Paul
Pedagogy of suffering, 180–81
Pennhurst, xiv, 117, 210–11
Pennsylvania Association for Retarded
　　Children (PARC), 56n3
"Perfect baby," expectations for, 111–13
Perinatal hospice, 226
Persistent vegetative state, 87, 187
Pervasive developmental disorder
　　(PDD), 141
Phases of care, 6, 74–93, 195, 222–23.
　　　See also Care-giving; Care-receiving;
　　　Caring about; Caring with; Taking
　　　care of
　　described, 78–93
　　social/political applications of, 77
Physical burden of care, 36–43
Physicians. See also Medical system
　　disagreements with, 127–28
　　second opinions discouraged
　　　by, 146–47
Pistorius, Martin, 34, 158–59
PKU, 211
Place for Noah, A (Greenfeld), 45
"Planet Autism" (Sea), xviii
*Plankton Dreams: What I Learned in
　　Special-Ed* (Mukhopadhyay), 168n1.
　　See also Tito
Pneumonia, 97, 101, 103, 127, 128, 187

Positive thinking. See Negativity silencing
Premature birth, 20, 23. See also Forman,
　　Ellie; Forman, Evan
　　grey zone, 67, 69
　　narrative of, 66–70
　　neonatology advances and, 27–28
　　quality of life and, 59–60
　　quest for knowledge on, 143
　　survival rates, 28
Prenatal screening, 117, 226. See also
　　Genetic testing
Presbyterian church, 203, 206, 207
Price, Beth, 195–96
Price, Jude (child with Down
　　syndrome), 195–96
Public Law 94-142, 56n3

Quality of life studies, 59–62
Quest narratives, 58–59, 134–56
　　facing failure, 148–56
　　level of knowledge obtained, 143–48
　　the search for information, 137–43

Rapid prompting method (RPM), 168n1
Rapp, Emily, 104, 112
　　ambivalence of, 109, 110
　　life story creation by, 162–63
　　quest for knowledge, 144
　　responsiveness and, 170–71, 178, 179, 184
Rapp, Ronan, 104, 109, 153, 162–63,
　　170–71, 178, 179, 184, 186, 226.
　　See also Rapp, Emily
Ray, Lynne, 15, 32, 38, 39, 42, 43, 48, 51,
　　52, 85, 93, 95, 98, 120, 130
Reciprocity, 87, 157. See also
　　Responsiveness
Redemptive narratives, 58
Respite care, 51, 131
Responsibility, 75, 76–77, 81–83, 94–123,
　　124, 126, 222
　　for advocacy (*see* Advocacy)
　　ambivalence and, 96, 103–10
　　attentiveness and, 83, 94–95
　　choice (perceived lack of) and,
　　　96, 116–21
　　extremes of, 81–82
　　uncertainty and, 96–103

Responsiveness, 75–77, 86–93, 94, 157–91
　care-receiver's responsibility in, 87–88
　the child as teacher of, 180–86
　to the child *vs.* the disease, 169–73
　consequences of lack of, 158
　extremes of, 89, 91–93
　feedback and, 84, 86–87, 91, 93, 157, 189
　hazards of, 163–69
　identity formation and life story creation in (*see* Identity; Life story)
　inquiring about needs, 157, 159
　letting go and, 186–91
　long-term care arrangements and, 213
　to nonverbal children, 173–80
Resuscitation
　legal requirement for, 66–67, 68
　of near-drowning victim, 96–97
　parents' attitudes toward, 69
　of premature babies, 28, 66–67, 68, 69
　of Trisomy18 infants, 29
Retinopathy of Prematurity (ROP), 143
Riding the Bus with My Sister (Simon), 34n2
Road Map to Holland (Groneberg), x

Saigal, Saroj, 59–60, 62
Samuel (child with CDLS), xvii–xviii
　current status of, 4, 226
　developmental level of, xvii
　financial burden of caring for, 49–50
　identity-disease interaction, 170, 171
　physical burden of caring for, 40–41, 43
Sandy (mother of individual with autism), 148–49, 153
Savannah (Savvy) (individual with CFC), 7, 168
　current status of, 4
　diagnosis of, 144
　life and development of, ix–xvi, 16–17, 20–21
　physical burden of caring for, 39–40, 43
　responsiveness and, 174–75, 179
Schomaker, Mary Zimmeth, 158
"School of Life, The" (Bremer), 136
Sea, S., xviii

Second opinions, discouragement of, 146–47
Seizures, 41, 71, 92–93, 132–33, 146. *See also* Forman, Evan; Lee, Lia
Selfhood, loss of, 79, 80, 91
Self-injurious behavior, 176
Self-stimulation (stimming), 164, 165
Sensory integration disorder, 141
Severe disability, 20, 28
Shame, 50–51, 52
Sheltered workshop system, 203–6
Sickle cell anemia, 91–92
Simon, Rachel, 34n2
60 Minutes (television program), 45
Slomka, Jacqueline, 69
Social isolation, 50–56
Social services, 51–52. *See also* Support systems and programs
Solidarity, as a virtue, 227–31
Solomon, Andrew, 25, 27
Soma (mother individual with autism), 164–68
Special needs. *See also* Children with special health care needs
　definition, 12–13, 21
　imprecision of term, 3, 10
Special Olympics, 195, 203, 206–7, 211
Specialness narrative, 113, 115
Spencer (child with special needs), 126–34, 135, 155
Spina bifida, 22, 117
Spink, Kathryn, 201–2
Spirit Catches You and You Fall Down, The (Fadiman), 41–42, 132–33. *See also* Fadiman, Anne; Lee, Fuoa; Lee, Lia
Stigmatization, 63, 96, 212, 213
Still Point of the Turning World, The (Rapp), 104. *See also* Rapp, Emily; Rapp, Ronin
Stimming. *See* Self-stimulation
Strange Son: Two Mothers, Two Sons, and the Quest to Unlock the Hidden World of Autism (Iversen), 164, 168. *See also* Iversen, Dov; Iversen, Portia; Soma; Tito
Suctioning, 16, 128, 129, 130–31, 133

Support systems and programs. *See also* Community
  improvement in availability of, 3–4
  inadequacy of, 51–52
  need for increase in, 155, 225–26

Taking care of (phase of care), 94, 124
  defined, 75
  process of, 81–83
  virtue associated with (*see* Responsibility)
Tax Equity Fairness and Responsibility Act, MN. *See* TEFRA
Tay-Sachs disease, 104, 112, 178, 226. *See also* Rapp, Ronan
  the child's identity and, 170–71
  life story creation and, 162–63
Technology dependence, 21–22, 34, 35
  competence in dealing with, 127–28
  defined, 15
  degree and types of, 24
  ethics literature on, 32
  financial burden of care and, 45, 46, 47
  parental vigilance and, 98
  physical burden of care and, 38–39
  prevalence of, 24
  social isolation and, 51
TEFRA, 24–26, 46, 47
"That Dragon, Cancer" (video game), 151
Theoretical-juridical model, 73
This Lovely Life (Forman), 66–73. *See also* Forman, Ellie; Forman, Evan; Forman, Vicky
Tito (individual with autism), 164–68. *See also* Mukhopadhyay, Tito
Toilet training, 40, 149. *See also* Diaper changes
Total dependency, 20
Tracheostomy, 39, 127, 128, 129, 130
Triest Hall, 215–19
Trisomy 18, 23, 28–29
Trisomy 21. *See* Down syndrome

Tronto, Joan, 4, 6, 66, 73–78, 81, 84, 86, 87, 88, 89, 94, 122, 124, 126, 129, 157, 185–86, 195, 222, 223, 226–27, 229, 230. *See also* Phases of care

Uncertainty, 96–103
Utter dependency, 11

Value, maintenance of, 110–16, 183–84, 209–10, 224
  gifts narrative and, 113–15
  specialness narrative and, 113, 115
Vanier, Jean, 195, 201–2, 213, 217, 220, 221
Velocardiofacial syndrome (VCFS), 53, 168
Ventilator dependence, 16, 32, 39, 118
Vigabitrin, 146
Vigilance, 98–99
Vineland Training School, 211
Virtue ethics, 73, 76, 223
Virtues, 74, 76. *See also* Attentiveness; Competence; Responsibility; Responsiveness
Visual impairment, 20, 22. *See also* Blindness; Retinopathy of Prematurity
Volbrecht, R. M., 84
Vulnerability, 86–87, 88

Walker, Margaret Urban, 73
"Welcome to Holland" (Kingsley), ix–xi, xiii–xiv, xv, xvi–xvii, xviii–xix, 1, 7, 9, 10, 30, 55, 111
Willowbrook State School, xiv, 210
Withholding treatment, xvii, 97, 101–3, 118, 187–89
Without Reason: A Family Copes with Two Generations of Autism (Hart), 50–51, 59, 106, 135. *See also* Hart, Charles; Hart, Ted
Wolf (child with VCFS), 168

Year of Magical Thinking, The (Didion), 144

Made in the USA
Monee, IL
03 May 2026

49437399R00151